# Breastfeeding
## the
## Late Preterm Infant

Praeclarus Press, LLC

2504 Sweetgum Lane

Amarillo, Texas 79124 USA

806-367-9950

www.PraeclarusPress.com

DISCLAIMER

The information contained in this publication is advisory only and is not intended to replace sound clinical judgment or individualized patient care. The author disclaims all warranties, whether expressed or implied, including any warranty as the quality, accuracy, safety, or suitability of this information for any particular purpose.

ISBN: 978-1-946665-47-8

Cover Design: Ken Tackett

Developmental Editing: Kathleen Kendall-Tackett

Copyediting: Chris Tackett

Layout & Design: Nelly Murariu

# Breastfeeding
## the
# Late Preterm Infant

Marsha Walker, RN, IBCLC

Praeclarus Press, LLC

*www.PraeclarusPress.com*

# Contents

## SECTION ONE      1

**Who is the Late Preterm Infant?**      3

Redefining Parental Expectations      3

Rate of Preterm Births in the U.S.      5

The Etiology of Late Preterm and Early Term Births      8

A Population at Risk      9

The Importance of the Last Six Weeks      14

Infant Brain Development      16

Cardiopulmonary System      20

Thermoregulation      21

Hypoglycemia      22

Hyperbilirubinemia (Jaundice)      24

**Perinatal Challenges**      26

Maternal Prenatal Medications      26

Labor Medications      27

Vacuum Extraction      29

Cesarean Delivery      30

Separation Immediately Following Delivery      31

Supplementation with a Feeding Bottle and Artificial Nipple      32

Delayed Lactogenesis II and Insufficient Milk Production      32

Maternal Conditions      34

**Parental Perceptions and Experiences of Breastfeeding a Late Preterm Infant**      35

# SECTION TWO

**SECTION TWO**     **39**

**Breastfeeding Management Guidelines**     **41**

**Getting Started with Breastfeeding**     **44**

    Skin-to-Skin Care     44

    Positioning     47

    Hypotonia and Immature Feeding Skills     49

    Latching and Latch Assistance     51

    The Latchable State     63

**Assessing Feedings at the Breast**     **67**

**Supplementation**     **69**

    Bottles     71

    Alternative Feeding Devices     72

**Feeding Plans**     **83**

    Hypoglycemia     86

**Initiating and Maintaining Maternal Milk Supply**     **91**

**Conclusion**     **96**

*Test Questions*     99

*Resources for Parents*     105

*Glossary*     107

*References*     113

*About the Author*     131

# SECTION ONE

# Who is the Late Preterm Infant?

There is a group of infants who historically were referred to as "slightly small," "mildly preterm," "just a little early," or "near term." These names describe a population of infants who may masquerade as large, healthy, and functional, while disguising their vulnerability to a host of medical and developmental challenges. They may be closer in appearance to term infants rather than extremely premature infants, making their unique vulnerabilities easy to overlook.

These babies are not just smaller versions of a full-term infant but are born during a period of rapid development and maturation of multiple organ and body systems. An abrupt halt to this in-utero maturation process can alter the eventual growth and development of the infant, as many organ systems have critical windows of time where certain events need to happen for a normal outcome. Even though late preterm infants may be born healthy, they remain at a much higher risk for a host of conditions that can compromise both breastfeeding and the infant's health.

Following a 2005 workshop convened by the National Institute of Child Health and Human Development (Raju et al., 2006), the designation "near term" was replaced with "late preterm." This was deemed a better descriptor of neonates who were at a higher risk than term infants for acute and chronic complications of prematurity. The committee expected that this change would better convey their greater vulnerabilities and need for closer monitoring and follow-up.

## Redefining Parental Expectations

Redefining this population of infants helps change the expectations of parents and clinicians of how these babies behave and how better to anticipate the type of care that they need. The panel also stated that gestational age should be rounded off to the nearest completed week, not to the following week. For example, clinicians would consider an infant born on the 4th day of the 35th week (35⁴) to be a gestational age of 35 weeks, not 36 weeks. Even infants born at 37 or 38 weeks are still physiologically immature and remain at a significantly higher risk for adverse outcomes.

In a study covering nearly 30,000 births it was found that adverse outcomes experienced by these early term babies (37 to 38 weeks) included hypoglycemia (4.9% versus 2.5% of full-term babies), admission to the neonatal intensive care unit (8.8% versus 5.3%), the need for respiratory support (2.0% versus 1.1%), the need for intravenous fluids (7.5% versus 4.4%) intravenous antibiotics (2.6% versus 1.6%), and mechanical ventilation or intubation, which was required in .6% of early term babies versus .1% in full-term babies.

The data also show that early term babies delivered by cesarean section were at a higher risk—by 12.2%—for admission to the NICU compared with full-term babies and at 7.5% higher risk for morbidity compared with term births (Sengupta et al., 2013). A study on gestational ages, birthweights, and obstetrical practices showed that between 1990 and 2013, the likelihood of induced labors and cesarean deliveries increased at all gestational ages, and the gestational age distribution of U.S. births shifted significantly. Births became much less likely to occur beyond 40 weeks of gestation and much more likely to occur during weeks 37–39 (early term infants). Overall, nearly 18% of births from not-induced labor and vaginal delivery at later gestational ages were replaced with births occurring at earlier gestational ages from obstetric interventions. Results of this study suggest that if rates of obstetric practices had not changed between 1990 and 2013, then the average U.S. birthweight would have increased during this time (Tilstra & Masters, 2020).

# Rate of Preterm Births in the U.S.

This issue is not likely to go away soon. The rate of premature birth in the United States increased 5% from 2014 (9.57%) to 2018 (10.02%), due primarily to the increase in late preterm births, which rose to 7.28% of all births (Figure 1). Late preterm births comprise over 70% of all preterm births (Figure 2). Non-Hispanic Black mothers have the highest late preterm birth rate of 9.23% compared with White mothers, who have a 6.83% late preterm birth rate (Hamilton et al., 2019).

**Figure 1.** Percentage of late preterm and early preterm births in the United States (Hamilton et al., 2019).

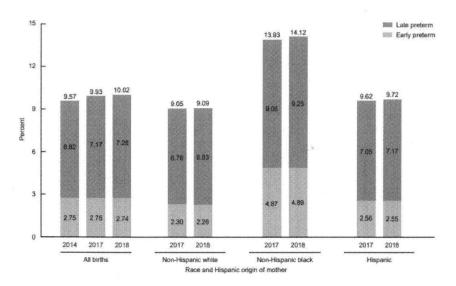

NOTE: Preterm is less than 37 weeks, late preterm is 34 to 36 weeks, and early preterm is less than 34 weeks of gestation.

SOURCE: NCHS, National Vital Statistics System, Natality.

**Figure 2.** Preterm birth breakdown for 2016 (Data from Martin JA, Hamilton BE, Osterman MJK, et al. Births: final data for 2016. Hyattsville (MD): U. S. Department of Health and Human Services; 2018.)

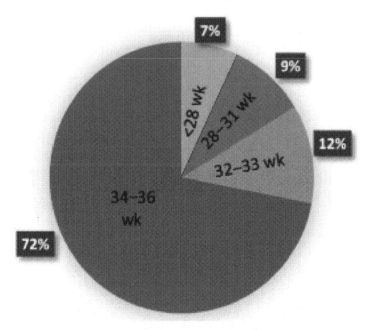

There are close to 400,000 preterm births annually in the U.S., approximately 280,000 of which are late preterm. In addition, several hundred thousand births occur each year between 37 and 38 weeks of gestation. These infants are called early term infants. Table 1 shows the nomenclature of prematurity (Rose & Engle, 2017).

Recognition of the health and developmental challenges that late preterm birth represents has resulted in public health efforts to reduce preterm birth and to provide clinicians with better tools to care for these infants. The Association for Women's Health, Obstetric, and Neonatal Nurses (AWHONN) created the Late Preterm Infant Initiative in 2005 as a multi-year endeavor to address the special needs of infants born between 34 and 36 completed weeks of gestation. The goals include increasing healthcare provider and consumer awareness of the risks associated with late preterm birth and ensuring evidence-based educational resources are available for nurses and healthcare providers to provide appropriate assessment and care for these vulnerable newborns. The March of Dimes Prematurity Campaign Collaborative launched in 2017, has 480 member organizations and over 700 individual members all working together to achieve equity and demonstrated improvements in preterm birth prevention. The Academy of Breastfeeding Medicine has developed a protocol for breastfeeding the late preterm and early term infant (Boies & Vaucher, 2016).

**Table 1.** The nomenclature of prematurity

| Weeks of gestation | Prematurity nomenclature |
|---|---|
| <37 weeks | |
| $<28^0$ weeks | Extremely preterm |
| $28^0$ to $31^6$ weeks | Very preterm |
| 32 to $33^6$ weeks | Moderately preterm |
| 34 to $36^6$ weeks | Late preterm |
| $37^0$ to $41^6$ weeks | Term |
| $37^0$ to $38^6$ weeks | Early term |
| $39^0$ to $41^6$ weeks | Full term |
| 42+ weeks | Post term |

The Federal government was concerned about the rising prematurity rates and in December 2006 congress passed the PREEMIE Act (P.L. 109-450) and renewed it in 2013. The act mandated an expansion in research, better provider education and training, and a Surgeon General's conference to address the growing epidemic of preterm births. This law was designed to improve the treatment and health of premature babies and to create programs to support the emotional and informational needs of their families. By reducing the number of babies who are born below normal birthweight, this legislation will help reduce healthcare costs for states, Medicaid, and other insurers. The law authorized a Surgeon General's conference at which scientific and clinical experts from the public and private sectors sat down together to formulate a national action agenda designed to speed development of prevention strategies for preterm labor and delivery. The PREEMIE Reauthorization Act of 2018 seeks renewal of the Federal government's commitment to preventing premature birth and its consequences.

## The Etiology of Late Preterm and Early Term Births

The etiology of late preterm and early term birth has a number of contributors (Brown et al., 2015; Delnord & Zeitlin, 2019) (Table 2) but in about half of spontaneous preterm births, the biological cause or pathogenesis is unknown (Ferrero et al., 2016; Stewart et al., 2019).

**Table 2.** Contributors to late preterm birth

| |
|---|
| Hypertension |
| Diabetes |
| Previous preterm or late preterm birth |
| Multiple pregnancy |
| Infection such as chorioamnionitis |
| Inflammation |
| Vascular disorders |
| Shortened cervix |
| Placental disorders |
| Medical indications |
| Adverse intrauterine environment<br>• Hypoxia<br>• Polyhydramnios<br>• Oligohydramnios |

# A Population at Risk

Late preterm infants are at an increased risk for airway instability, cardio-respiratory instability, apnea, bradycardia, excessive sleepiness, large weight loss, dehydration, feeding difficulties, weak sucking, jaundice, hypoglycemia, hypothermia, immature self-regulation, respiratory distress, sepsis, prolonged formula supplementation, hospital re-admission, and breastfeeding failure during the neonatal period (Natarajan & Shankaran, 2016). The younger the baby, the higher the risk. Late preterm infants are at risk for acute morbidities starting immediately following delivery and extending well into childhood (Table 3) (Huff, Rose, & Engle, 2019).

Respiratory issues are more common in late preterm infants because the pulmonary system is one of the last fetal organ systems to mature. Fetal lungs are filled with fluid that must be cleared for adequate gas exchange to occur following birth. In late gestation, and as labor progresses, the production of lung fluid decreases and transporters in the lungs that increase lung fluid clearance are induced, so that lung fluid can be cleared rapidly. Synthesis of surfactant and antioxidant enzymes also increases towards the end of pregnancy to prepare the lungs for air breathing.

Hormonal and physiological changes associated with labor are necessary for lung maturation in neonates. These changes may be altered or interrupted in cesarean deliveries because of pulmonary immaturity and the lack of beneficial effects of normal labor on the newborn. These effects include the reduction in lung fluid, enhanced catecholamine levels, secretion of surfactant stores into the alveolar space, and increased levels of pulmonary vasodilating substances.

**Table 3.** Morbidity and mortality among late preterm infants (Huff, Rose, & Engle, 2019).

| Condition | Increased Risk Compared with Term Infants |
|---|---|
| Resuscitation at delivery | 46% vs. 28% |
| Temperature instability | 10% |
| Feeding difficulties | 32% vs. 7% |
| Increased time to full oral feedings | Median time:<br>12 days at 34 weeks<br>3 days at 35 weeks<br>2 days at 36 weeks |
| Longer length of birth hospitalization | Average time:<br>12.6 days at 34 weeks<br>6.1 days at 35 weeks<br>3.8 days at 36 weeks |
| Most common factors leading to increased length of stay | Feeding difficulties 75.9%<br>Respiratory distress 30.8%<br>Jaundice 16.3% |
| Developmental delay<br>Cognitive dysfunction/cerebral palsy | 12/1000 at 34 weeks<br>9/1000 at 34 weeks<br>9/1000 at 38-41 weeks<br>3/1000 at 38-41 weeks |
| Respiratory syncytial virus hospitalization during the first 2 years after birth | 2.5% vs. 1.3% |
| Mortality | Per 1000 live births<br>7.23 from 34-36 weeks<br>3.01 from 37-38 weeks<br>1.85 for 39-40 weeks |

Maternal factors can contribute to an increased incidence of sepsis or infection in late preterm infants. Chorioamnionitis (inflammation/infection of the membranes and chorion of the placenta) and premature rupture of the membranes may contribute not only to the etiology of preterm labor, but may also be implicated in the higher incidence of respiratory infection seen in late preterm infants (McDowell et al., 2016). Delayed lung maturation and increased risk of respiratory distress syndrome have been consistently observed among infants born to mothers with diabetes (Azad et al., 2017). Cesarean delivery not only negatively affects the benefits of normal labor on the pulmonary transition to air breathing, but late preterm delivery and cesarean section also alter the infant gut microbiota that can lead to infant gut dysbiosis (perturbations in gut bacterial balance).

## Infant Gut Microbiome

Early infant bacterial gut colonization and composition exerts a significant impact on health and disease with specific members of the infant gut microbiota implicated in the subsequent development of atopic disease, allergy, autoimmune diseases, autism spectrum disorders, and metabolic disease including overweight and obesity (Rautava et al., 2012). Even though the gut microbiome is negatively altered by cesarean delivery and maternal and neonatal antibiotic use, late preterm birth independently affects gut microbiota development, which differs significantly from that of full-term infants (Forsgren et al., 2017).

One type of bacterium in particular, the Bifidobacterium genus, helps the infant gut to be more resistant to colonization by pathogens, respond better to some vaccines, possess better gut barrier function, and reduce inflammation (Fukuda et al., 2011; Huda, et al., 2014; Romond, et al., 2008). Bifidobacteria are reduced in the presence of late preterm birth and are further depleted by cesarean delivery, maternal and infant antibiotic use, and formula feeding rather than breastfeeding.

Bifidobacteria use the oligosaccharides in breastmilk as a food source in order to proliferate, enhance intestinal epithelial cell function, and maintain a balance between pathologic and non-pathologic gut bacteria (Chichlowski, et al., 2012).

Some late preterm infants may take weeks to acquire competent breastfeeding skills, during which time the mother's milk supply is at risk unless regular milk expression is initiated to compensate until the infant can demonstrate adequate milk transfer. If the mother is not producing sufficient milk for infant growth, the use of banked donor human milk or infant formula supplementation may be necessary until milk production matches infant needs. Some mothers may also have other risk factors for insufficient milk, which compound this problem (preterm delivery itself, cesarean delivery, overweight or obesity, endocrine problems, delayed lactogenesis II, insufficient pumping).

In an analysis of 802 late preterm infants, Medoff-Cooper and colleagues found that late preterm infants of all gestational ages were most likely to be fed by a combination of breastmilk and formula, with feeding difficulties identified in 40.6% of the infants (Medoff-Cooper et al., 2012). The occurrence of some of the conditions experienced by late preterm, as well as early term infants, may be exacerbated by initial caretaking behaviors following delivery. In the Medoff-Cooper study, 32% of the infants were bathed during the first 2 hours of life and by 4 hours, more than two thirds had had their first bath. Also seen was 48% of the infants receiving no skin-to-skin care during the first 48 hours of life—both of which contribute to hypoglycemia and temperature instability.

## Hospital Readmission Rates

Hospital readmission rates for late preterm infants are 1.5 to 3 times that of full-term infants (Kuzniewicz, et al., 2013). The most frequent reasons for readmission are sepsis, jaundice, and feeding problems.

In an evaluation of 1,683 late-preterm and 33,745 term infants, researchers found that the average length of stay of the birth hospitalization for term infants was 2.2 days, and the average cost was $2,061. Late-preterm infants had a significantly longer average stay of 8.8 days with an average cost of $26,054. Total first-year costs after birth discharge were, on average, three times as high among late-preterm infants ($12,247) compared with term infants ($4,069). Late-preterm infants were re-hospitalized more often than term infants (15.2% vs. 7.9%) (McLaurin et al., 2009).

In somewhat of a paradox, re-admission of breastfed late preterm infants is nearly twice as common as re-admission of formula-fed late preterm infants or breastfed term infants (Radtke, 2011). Even though breastfeeding and the provision of human milk is optimal for this population, feeding-related problems of jaundice, weight loss, and dehydration are seen in many late preterm infants, as well as some early term infants whose ability to successfully transfer sufficient amounts of breastmilk is compromised.

## Policy Regarding Late Preterm Birth

Recognizing the gravity of late preterm birth, the American College of Obstetricians and Gynecologists (ACOG) issued a Committee Opinion on reducing the number of late preterm and early term deliveries by recommending that timing of elective delivery should be at 39 weeks or later (American College of Obstetricians and Gynecologists, 2019a) unless an earlier delivery is warranted due to maternal or fetal complications (American College of Obstetricians and Gynecologists, 2019b). The timing of delivery in such cases must balance the maternal and infant risks of late preterm and early term birth with the risks associated with continuation of the pregnancy. If a late preterm delivery is anticipated (versus a spontaneous late preterm birth), ACOG recommends that a single course of betamethasone be administered within 7 days of delivery to accelerate fetal lung maturity.

Infants mature at different rates in utero, just as their individual organ systems follow a maturational path. Even though infants may be "safely" delivered prior to their due date, size and weight are not indications of maturity. While all the organ systems have formed, their final maturation occurs during the last stage of pregnancy, preparing the infant for life outside the support of the womb. Infants born early have limited compensatory mechanisms to adjust rapidly to the extra-uterine environment. Infants who miss the last six weeks of pregnancy are born with multiple vulnerabilities that compromise their health, as well as their ability to breastfeed.

## The Importance of the Last Six Weeks

The last four to six weeks of pregnancy is a critical maturational period for the fetus. It represents a period of rapid brain growth and matura-tion of body and organ systems. Glycogen stores increase in the liver (a source of glucose to maintain blood sugar levels immediately following birth), subcutaneous tissue and brown fat stores develop (a source of energy), muscle tone increases, and an increased passage of maternal antibodies through the placenta is seen. Iron stores are transferred from mother to infant during this period as well and, if missed, the infant is at higher risk for anemia which can have unwanted neurode-velopmental effects. The brain experiences a five-fold increase in white matter and a 33% growth in brain volume during this time (Bennett et al., 2018). Interruption of these maturational processes leaves the late preterm and early term infant physiologically, metabolically, and neurologically immature with limited compensatory mechanisms to adjust to the extrauterine environment and perform the tasks neces-sary to successfully breastfeed.

### Neurological System

At birth, the brain mass of 34 to 35 week late preterm infants is approximately 60% that of term infants, myelination is markedly underdeveloped, and neuronal connections and synaptic junctions are not fully developed (Figure 3).

**Figure 3.** Brain development and striking difference between the brain of a 36-week fetus and one who has reached 40 weeks. (Source: Volpe, Neurology of the Newborn, 3rd Ed, 1995.)

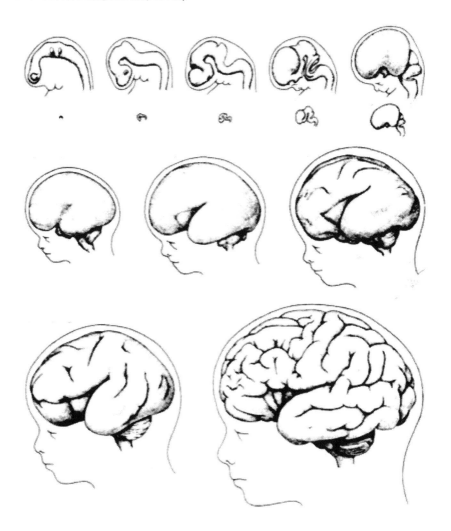

## Infant Brain Development

As the billions of nerve cells (neurons) are formed in the brain over the 40 weeks of gestation, there are many critical events that occur during this development, one of which is myelination. Myelin is a fatty substance that coats the axons (branches of the nerve cell), acts as an electrical insulator, and is vital to information flow along the neuron. Myelin's most important function is to speed the transmission of electrical signals, which is accomplished by the flow of ions (dissolved salts like sodium, calcium, potassium, and chloride). However, nerve cells are leaky and as electrical signals speed along the length of an axon, some of the ions leak out, reducing the efficiency of the transmission. Myelination prevents this from happening by laying down a sealing coat of material that keeps ions from leaking.

Myelination begins in the second trimester of pregnancy and continues into adult life. Myelination in the brain begins before birth within the caudal brain stem and progresses rostrally to the forebrain, with the most rapid and dramatic period of human central myelination within the first two years of postnatal life. It is during this critical period that myelin is initially laid down in virtually all white-matter tracts. Because myelin contains an abundant amount of fat, it has a white appearance, thus the term white matter is applied.

The brain of a late preterm or early term infant is not simply a smaller version of a term infant's brain. The brain of the late preterm and early term infant has experienced an interruption in development and must perform tasks for which it may not yet be maturationally ready. The physiologic maturity to accomplish a coordinated and effective suck/swallow/breath pattern occurs right at the time late preterm infants are born (Hallowell & Spatz, 2012). Breastmilk essentially assumes the extrauterine role of brain building by providing the substrates of the intrauterine environment. Deoni and colleagues (2013) found that when compared to formula-fed infants, breastfed infants had several advantages in terms of brain development.

- They showed enhanced brain growth of 20% to 30%.

- By age 2, infants exclusively breastfed for at least three months had enhanced development in key parts of the brain compared to children who were fed formula exclusively, or who were fed a combination of formula and breastmilk. The extra growth was most pronounced in parts of the brain associated with language, emotional function, and cognition.

- Infants who were breastfed for more than a year compared with those breastfed less than a year, had significantly enhanced brain growth especially in areas of the brain dealing with motor function.

- Infants who were exclusively breastfed had the fastest growth in myelinated white matter compared with formula-fed infants, with the increase in white matter volume becoming substantial by age 2.

The neural control of breathing and respiratory rhythm is in the brainstem. Brainstem respiratory centers provide the neural drive for upper airway muscles that maintain airway patency and control contractions of the diaphragm, intercostal, and laryngeal muscles, which carry out the physical tasks of breathing movements. An immature brainstem can adversely affect arousal, sleep-wake behavior, and the coordination of feeding with breathing.

Late preterm infants are at increased risk for lower general cognitive ability, lower IQ, developmental delay, poorer language and school performance, increased special education needs, increased utilization of early intervention services, and a higher risk for teacher-reported behavioral problems (Chan et al., 2016; Woythaler, 2019). Because brain growth and development occurs in a very specific order and time frame, as well as at different rates, injury or insults (such as preterm birth, jaundice, hypoglycemia) happening during a critical period of growth could change the trajectory of brain development. Simply being born preterm has been shown to alter brain growth, as evidenced by differences seen in magnetic resonance imaging between late preterm and full-term infants (Walsh et al., 2014).

## The Importance of Breastmilk for Brain Growth and Maturation of the Late Preterm Infant

Human milk for preterm infants of any gestational age is vital to the optimal development of a brain that has been challenged by an early birth. Breastfeeding and/or the provision of breastmilk have been associated with improved developmental growth in late maturing white matter brain regions. Extended breastfeeding duration is associated with improved white matter structure and cognitive performance compared with formula-fed infants. This may be due to the specific brain-enhancing components found in breastmilk, such as the long-chain polyunsaturated fatty acids, docosahexanoic acid (DHA) and arachidonic acid (ARA), and cholesterol and nerve growth factors.

A study of low birthweight preterm infants found that cerebral white matter showed significantly greater levels of inositol (a molecule similar to glucose) for babies fed breast milk, compared with babies fed formula. Cerebellar areas had significantly greater creatine levels for breastfed babies compared with infants fed formula, and the percentage of days infants were fed breastmilk was associated with significantly greater levels of both creatine and choline, a water-soluble nutrient (Ottolini et al., 2019).

Greater quantities of creatine denotes more rapid changes and higher cellular maturation. Choline is a marker of cell membrane turnover. When new cells are generated, choline levels rise. Breastmilk naturally contains sphingomyelin, an important structural component of myelin that is absent in infant formula. These substances, as well as others, may promote preferential neural growth and white matter development (Deoni et al., 2013) (Table 4).

**Table 4.** Selected human milk components that support brain development compared with infant formula

| Human milk component | Function |
|---|---|
| Sialic acid | Essential component of brain gangliosides that are involved in cell-to-cell interaction, neuronal outgrowth, synaptic connectivity, and memory formation. Infant formula contains <25% of sialic acid compared with human milk, one form of which is implicated in some human inflammatory diseases (Wang, 2009). |
| Lactose (galactose+glucose) | The presence of abundant amounts of galactose helps assure an adequate supply of galactocerebrosides to the brain needed for myelination. Infants fed formulas with no lactose, such as soy formulas or cow's milk-based formula with the lactose removed, consume a diet lacking in brain growth nutrients. |
| Antioxidant capacity | Total antioxidant capacity is significantly higher in breastmilk than formula, conferring better protection against necrotizing enterocolitis, retinopathy of prematurity, chronic lung disease, intraventricular hemorrhage (brain bleed), and periventricular leukomalacia (softening and death of brain tissue;) (Aycicek et al., 2006). |
| Human milk oligosaccharide 2'-fucosyllactose (2'FL) | The amount of 2'FL in breast milk in the first month of feeding was related to significantly higher cognitive development scores in babies by 2 years of age. The amount of 2'FL in breast milk at six months of feeding was not related to cognitive outcomes, indicating that early exposure may be more beneficial (Berger et al., 2020). |

| | |
|---|---|
| Docosahexaenoic acid (DHA) and arachidonic acid (AA) | DHA and AA added to infant formula are sourced from fermented microalgae and soil fungus and are not structurally the same. No clear evidence has been found that formula supplementation with DHA/AA improves infant brain development when compared to breastfed infants (Jasani et al., 2017) |

## Cardiopulmonary System

Late preterm infants are at a greater risk for lung morbidities because they are born during a period when alveoli are maturing, surfactant levels are increasing, and the lungs are changing from fluid secretion organs to fluid absorption organs. Birth prior to lung maturation delays amniotic fluid clearance, reduces maintenance of alveolar expansion, and decreases lung perfusion. It places these infants at risk for respiratory distress syndrome, transient tachypnea, bradycardia, persistent pulmonary hypertension, and respiratory failure. Cesarean birth in the absence of labor further exacerbates these conditions.

Apnea occurs more frequently in late preterm infants, affecting up to 10% of those born at 34 and 35 weeks (Zhao et al., 2011). Late preterm infants may be less sensitive to higher levels of carbon dioxide and may experience decreased upper airway dilator muscle tone (Engle et al., 2007). They may also be at increased risk for centrally mediated apnea because their central nervous systems are developmentally immature, with fewer sulci and gyri in the brain and less myelin. Late preterm infants have approximately twice the risk for sudden infant death syndrome (Ostfeld et al., 2017).

Congenital heart disease and patent ductus arteriosis are more common in late preterm infants and may further compromise feeding issues and weight gain. Some infants with heart anomalies may not only feed poorly and tire out prior to the completion of a feeding, but may also demonstrate sweating while feeding, develop rapid breathing (tachypnea) and a rapid heart rate (tachycardia), or show circumoral cyanosis.

Young adults who were born premature have been shown to have alterations in the characteristics of their hearts, such as smaller heart chambers and higher blood pressure. This may manifest as an increased risk for cardiovascular incidents, high blood pressure, and reduced exercise tolerance. However, the smaller heart chambers were less profound for an exclusively human milk-fed group in comparison to those who were exclusively formula-fed as infants, suggesting a potentially protective effect of human milk for heart structure. Early exposure to breast milk may slow down or even arrest those pathophysiological changes, thereby mitigating the long-term adverse effects of premature birth on cardiovascular health (El-Khuffash et al., 2019).

## Thermoregulation

Temperature instability is a common problem in late preterm infants. Brown fat stores, maturation of the processes needed to mobilize these stores, and hormones involved in brown fat metabolism do not peak until term (Stephenson et al., 2001; Symonds et al., 2003). When activated at birth from the cold challenge of the extrauterine environment, brown adipose tissue can generate a significant amount of heat. Brown adipose tissue usually comprises 2% to 4% of birthweight, with term infants also possessing a substantial amount of white adipose tissue that helps as an insulation mechanism. In preterm infants, there can be a disruption in the switching on of brown adipose tissue that impairs heat production and can result in hypothermia (Symonds, 2013). Preterm infants possess less subcutaneous fat for insulation, their skin is a poor barrier to evaporative heat loss, and they may draw against limited glycogen stores in the liver to generate heat resulting in a quick depletion of glucose and the development of hypoglycemia.

Cold stress in late preterm infants is a significant factor leading to poor initiation of breastfeeding and the development of hypoglycemia (Laptook & Jackson, 2006). Newborn infants receive a bath early in the neonatal period to decrease the transmission of communicable diseases via blood and body fluid contact. The first bath is thought to be necessary to prevent cross contamination of body fluids between the newborn and the healthcare provider. Infants were traditionally given a sponge bath because it was thought to decrease the risk of infection prior to umbilical cord detachment.

Immersion tub bathing, when compared to sponge bathing, however, has been shown to result in improved thermoregulation in the late preterm infant following the bathing procedure (Loring et al., 2012). Many hospitals delay newborn bathing for 12 to 24 hours when newborns are at the greatest risk for complications related to cold stress, such as hypoglycemia, respiratory distress, poor tone, and tachypnea. DiCioccio and colleagues (2019) demonstrated that delaying the newborn bath was also associated with increased in-hospital exclusive breastfeeding rates.

## Hypoglycemia

At birth, the newborn's glucose concentration is approximately 80% of maternal glucose, but it declines rapidly to its lowest level between 30 and 90 minutes after birth and stabilizes between 40 to 100 mg/dL by 4 hours after birth (Committee on Fetus and Newborn, 2011). Once the cord is clamped, the newborn must adapt swiftly in order to produce endogenous glucose to meet the energy demands of cellular oxidation. During this transition, the newborn infant's circulating glucose concentration decreases to one third of the maternal concentration (40 to 60 mg/dL) by 2 to 4 hours of age. In the late premature infant, this concentration may drop even lower at 30 to 40 mg/dL.

Late preterm infants are at a higher risk for hypoglycemia due to their diminished liver glycogen stores and immature hepatic energy pathways. Their counterregulatory efforts are less efficient, as they have difficulty generating glucose until their metabolic pathways can compensate. Alternate fuels, such as lactate, pyruvate, amino acids, free fatty acids, ketone bodies, and glycerol are used by the brain during hypoglycemia. Unlike term infants, however, late preterm infants have difficulty mounting an adequate mature peripheral counter-regulatory ketogenic response to hypoglycemia. This is because of inadequate lipolysis in these infants who do not have the necessary adipose tissue stores and may fail to demonstrate adequate milk intake (Garg & Devaskar, 2006). They can also be affected by other stressors, such as sepsis, crying, perinatal stress, cesarean delivery, and cold stress that further contribute to hypoglycemia.

The American Academy of Pediatrics (AAP) published clinical management guidelines on Postnatal Glucose Homeostasis in Late-Preterm and Term Infants (Committee on Fetus and Newborn, 2011). The Academy of Breastfeeding Medicine (ABM) has also published Guidelines for Blood Glucose Monitoring and Treatment of Hypoglycemia in Term and Late-Preterm Neonates (Wight et al., 2014).

Hyperinsulinism may be encountered in infants of diabetic mothers, and in babies whose mothers have a high BMI and are insulin resistant. This happens because glucose freely passes into the placenta from the maternal circulation, and the neonatal pancreas responds by increasing insulin secretion and becoming hypertrophied. On delivery, the maternal glucose supply stops, and it takes time for the neonatal pancreas to adjust. It can cause significant hypoglycemia, but normally resolves in a period of days. Transient hyperinsulinism, also inactivates the usual counter-regulatory responses (glycogenolysis, gluconeogenesis, lipolysis, and β-oxidation of fatty acids) to loss of glucose supply from the placenta and increases peripheral glucose utilization further contributing to hypoglycemia.

## Hyperbilirubinemia (Jaundice)

Jaundice is one of the leading causes of re-hospitalization in late preterm infants. Experience and reports indicate that the morbidity rate due to hyperbilirubinemia doubles for each week less than 39 weeks of gestation (Bhutani, 2012). Jaundice and hyperbilirubinemia occur more commonly, and are more prolonged, among late preterm infants than term infants. The American Academy of Pediatrics (AAP) published clinical management guidelines on hyperbilirubinemia, which contain a nomogram for risk designation of newborns based on hour-specific serum bilirubin values (American Academy of Pediatrics, Subcommittee on Hyperbilirubinemia, 2004).

Infants born at 35 to 36 weeks are at a high risk for hyperbilirubinemia. Those born at 37 to 38 weeks demonstrate a moderate risk. And infants born at 39 weeks and beyond are placed in the low-risk category. Bilirubin levels in late preterm infants peak later (at seven rather than at five days), stay elevated for longer, and reach higher mean values compared with term infants. The late preterm infant is probably at risk of kernicterus at lower levels of bilirubin than the term infant (Whyte et al., 2010). This occurs due to slower meconium passage, decreased activity of the bilirubin-conjugating enzyme uridine diphosphate glucuronyl transferase (UGT), and low breastmilk intake.

Exclusive breastfeeding increases the risk of extreme hyperbilirubinemia by a factor of approximately six (Whyte et al., 2010). Breastfeeding difficulties predispose late preterm infants to an increase in enterohepatic circulation of bilirubin due to decreased stool frequency, reduced caloric intake, increased weight loss, dehydration, and hypernatremia that add to the overall bilirubin burden and risk of toxicity. The slow passage of meconium presents a greater opportunity for the bilirubin reservoir to re-enter the infant's circulation and contribute to continuously rising bilirubin levels that exaggerates jaundice in this population.

Poor breastfeeding can consist of a number of indicators, such as failure to latch, poor latch that does not transfer adequate colostrum or breastmilk, weak sucking pressures, lack of documented swallowing, inability to sustain nutritive sucking long enough to ingest a sufficient volume of colostrum/breastmilk, and excessive sleepiness that leaves late preterm infants underfed. Interventions to support adequate milk transfer or in its absence sufficient expressed colostrum/breastmilk intake are vital to prevent prolonged hospital stays and readmission shortly after hospital discharge.

Other clinical factors may further contribute to rising bilirubin levels, such as race/ethnicity (East Asian, Native American), degree of immaturity, bruising, blood group incompatibility, G6PD deficiency, cephalohematoma, vacuum delivery, certain maternal medications, such as oxytocin and diazepam, and infant vulnerabilities to inherent, familial or genetic co-morbidities. Climbing bilirubin levels at any gestational age signal the need for increased vigilance and more intensive lactation support.

# Perinatal Challenges

In addition to the immaturity of multiple systems in the late preterm infant, events, situations, and interventions during the peripartum period can pose even more challenges to breastfeeding. Some families experience multiple simultaneous challenges that further complicate both breastfeeding and lactation.

## Maternal Prenatal Medications

Fetal exposure to certain maternal antidepressive medications can affect feeding ability and other neurological parameters in neonates. A meta-analysis suggested that neonates exposed to maternal antidepressants during pregnancy were five times more likely to experience transient neonatal adaptation symptoms than non-exposed neonates (Grigoriadis et al., 2013). Transient adverse neonatal signs and symptoms such as respiratory distress, tremors, irritability, hypotonia, and poor feeding may affect up to 30% of newborns exposed to selective serotonin reuptake inhibitors (SSRIs) (Grigoriadis et al., 2013; Rampono et al., 2009). SSRIs are medications, such as sertraline (Zoloft), fluoxetine (Prozac), venlafaxine (Effexor), and citalopram (Celexa).

Even lower tone was found in SSRI-exposed infants with concomitant benzodiazepine (e.g., diazepam (Valium) exposure). These infants had the lowest movement quality scores and highest number of CNS stress signs extending beyond the first 7 to 10 days postpartum (Salisbury et al., 2016). Concomitant use of benzodiazepines in conjunction with SSRIs was associated with more significant problems in infant neurological functioning than SSRI use alone (Salisbury et al., 2016). Clinicians will need to provide extra vigilance in regard to infant breastfeeding behaviors, milk transfer, and neonatal weight gain for late preterm infants who have been exposed to these drugs.

Maternal receipt of antenatal corticosteroids (such as betamethasone) to reduce infant short-term respiratory morbidity can increase and exacerbate neonatal hypoglycemia (Groom, 2019).

## Labor Medications

The ability of a late preterm infant to successfully breastfeed may be impeded by maternal labor medications. Nalbuphine (Nubain) is a synthetic opioid analgesic that, if used during labor, could have potential side effects on the newborn. Fetal and neonatal adverse effects that have been reported following the administration of nalbuphine to the mother during labor include fetal bradycardia, respiratory depression at birth, apnea, cyanosis, and hypotonia (Food and Drug Administration, 2016). The risk for hypotonia (low muscle tone) is of particular concern, as normal muscle tone is necessary for the lips to maintain a seal on the breast, for the jaw and tongue to work in a coordinated manner, and for a high enough vacuum to be exerted to initiate and maintain milk flow from the breast.

Pre-feeding cues exhibited by infants are oral-motor neurobehaviors that indicate feeding readiness and behavioral state control. Intrapartum synthetic oxytocin is commonly used for labor induction and augmentation. In a study sample of 47 healthy full-term infants (36 exposed to synthetic oxytocin and 11 infants not exposed), fewer pre-feeding cues were observed in infants exposed to synthetic oxytocin. Forty-four percent of exposed infants demonstrated a low level of pre-feeding organization compared to none from the unexposed group. Exposed infants were 11.5 times more likely to exhibit low pre-feeding organization compared to unexposed infants (Bell et al., 2013).

Lactate is a byproduct of muscle activity, including the uterine muscle. Levels of lactate in amniotic fluid increase during labor, more so in deliveries where synthetic oxytocin is used. Increased stimulation of the uterine contractions with synthetic oxytocin may cause an even more excessive uterine production of lactate under conditions where its removal is impaired.

A study looked at the level of lactate in amniotic fluid and its association with the use of synthetic oxytocin and adverse neonatal outcomes. In the group with adverse neonatal outcomes, which included fetal hypoxia (lack of oxygen), the level of lactate in amniotic fluid was significantly higher in the final sample before delivery compared to the group with lower levels of lactate. The frequency of adverse neonatal outcomes was associated with the level of lactate in amniotic fluid and with the use of synthetic oxytocin, with more neonatal adverse outcomes experienced the higher the levels of lactate rose (Wiberg-Itzel et al., 2014). Hypoxia can adversely affect sucking and swallowing (Slattery et al., 2012), resulting in more feeding difficulties in already compromised infants.

Intrapartum exposure to both fentanyl in epidural analgesia and synthetic oxytocin significantly decreased the likelihood of a newborn infant suckling while skin-to-skin with the mother during the first hour post birth (Brimdyr et al., 2015). The mean amount of fentanyl that mothers received in this study without receipt of synthetic oxytocin was 169.64 mcg, while mothers who received fentanyl with synthetic oxytocin received a mean of 264.45 mcg. An inverse relationship was seen between the dose of fentanyl and infant suckling in the first hour post birth.

As the dose of fentanyl increased, the likelihood of successful suckling decreased. There was a stepwise decrease in the proportion of infant suckling within the first hour beginning at approximately a 150-mcg dose of fentanyl. Beilin et al. (2005) showed that infants of women who received >150 micrograms of fentanyl during labor had lower neurobehavioral scores after birth and decreased breastfeeding duration at 6 weeks postpartum (Beilin et al., 2005).

Widstrom et al. (2011) documented nine stages of instinctive behavior that newborns engage in while skin-to-skin during the first hour post birth. These range from the birth cry, through crawling to the breast and suckling, to falling asleep. Infants who were exposed to both fentanyl and synthetic oxytocin were less likely to progress through these stages, culminating in failure to seek and attach to the breast during the first hour compared with infants who were not exposed (Brimdyr et al., 2019).

Under the influence of fentanyl and synthetic oxytocin, attaching and sucking at the breast is reduced during this unique and sensitive period. Early successful initiation of breastfeeding during the first hour after birth is associated with achieving exclusive breastfeeding intentions (Perrine et al., 2012). Intrapartum administration of fentanyl and synthetic oxytocin present another challenge to the late preterm infant and serve as an indication for closer lactation-related monitoring and follow-up.

## Vacuum Extraction

Labor medications may increase the risk of assisted birth. Epidural analgesia is a risk factor for the use of vacuum extraction (Hasegawa et al., 2013). In 2017, there were almost 97,000 U.S. births assisted by vacuum extraction (Martin et al., 2019). Vacuum-assisted vaginal deliveries can cause significant fetal morbidity, including scalp lacerations, cephalohematomas, subgaleal hematomas, intracranial hemorrhage, facial nerve palsies, hyperbilirubinemia, and retinal hemorrhage (Ali & Norwitz, 2009). Late preterm infants can suffer more complications from vacuum extraction, such as scalp edema, bone fracture, and cephalohematomas compared with full term infants (Simonson et al., 2007). Hall et al. (2002) demonstrated that vacuum extraction was a strong predictor of breastfeeding cessation by 7 to 10 days.

## Cesarean Delivery

Mothers delivering by cesarean section have reported more problems with latching, positioning, and more pain when compared to women experiencing a vaginal birth (Brown & Jordan, 2013).

Postoperative pain is not limited to the immediate postpartum period, as women who have undergone a cesarean section may report problems with pain for as long as 4 to 8 weeks after the surgery (Schytt et al., 2005). Pain and stress have long been known to inhibit the milk-ejection reflex (Newton & Newton, 1948), which may limit the amount of milk a baby receives at each feeding.

Only small volumes of milk (1mL to 10 mL) can be expressed (Kent et al., 2003) or obtained by the breastfeeding infant (Ramsay et al., 2004) prior to activation of the milk- ejection reflex. A late preterm infant may simply not possess the stamina to sustain sucking until the milk-ejection reflex occurs or be too fatigued to feed once it does.

Lactogenesis II may be equally affected by the insult of abdominal surgery in both planned and emergency cesarean sections, with a delay in the onset of copious milk production (Dewey et al., 2003). This may result in a prolonged colostral phase whereby colostrum may be present for 4 to 5 days rather than transitioning to mature milk and increasing in volume by 72 hours as in a vaginal delivery.

Limitations on milk volume may predispose the late preterm infant to an even higher risk of weight loss, dehydration, hypoglycemia, and jaundice. Lactogenesis II can also be delayed in the presence of maternal diabetes (DeBortoli & Amir, 2016) and a high body mass index (BMI) (Turcksin et al., 2014). The combination of a cesarean delivery of a late preterm infant to a mother with a high BMI and diabetes presents a high-risk situation for poor breastfeeding outcomes.

# Separation Immediately Following Delivery

The act of separation itself can result in reduced blood glucose levels, adding an additional risk of hypoglycemia to an infant already prone to developing low blood glucose levels immediately following birth. Newborn infants who were immediately separated from their mothers, swaddled, and placed in a bassinet were shown to have decreased temperature and blood glucose levels compared to infants who were kept skin to skin (Christensson et al., 1992; Mazurek et al., 1999). Separating newborns from their mother increases cortisol levels, placing infants under stress that could result in alterations in neurodevelopment and unwelcome epigenetic changes (Csaszar-Nagy & Bokkon, 2018).

Babies cry when separated from their mother because of the absence of the maternal sensory regulators (Hofer, 2005). This shuts off the baby's growth hormone and switches on cortisol (Hofer, 1994). Cortisol diverts calories and other neurological resources such that homeostasis is re-established, but at the cost of growth. Such infants may have stable vital signs, but calories are consumed to achieve this homeostasis (McEwen & Seeman, 1999).

When the mother provides regulation through her own body, the baby's energy is available for development. In a study of two-day-old healthy babies sleeping alternatively in a bassinet and in skin-to-skin care (their own controls), bassinet sleeping showed three times higher autonomic nervous system (ANS) activation compared with skin to skin (Morgan, Horn, & Bergman, 2011).

More calories are required with higher ANS activity, which is accompanied by high cortisol levels. When cortisol is doing the regulating, less efficient homeostatic set-points are being programmed in the physiology of the baby. This unnecessary burning of calories can contribute to not only hypoglycemia but also to hyperbilirubinemia and weight loss. For the infant, the promotion of Zero Separation is based on the need for maternal sensory inputs that regulate the physiology of the newborn (Bergman, 2014).

## Supplementation with a Feeding Bottle and Artificial Nipple

If a late preterm infant requires supplemental feeding, it is often provided with a feeding bottle and artificial nipple. It has long been known that bottle-feeding infants may exhibit lower oxygen saturation levels than breastfeeding infants, experience periods of actual oxygen desaturation during feeding, develop bradycardia, and show a higher rate of swallowing and increased interruptions in breathing while feeding from a bottle (Meier, 1988; Thoyre & Carlson, 2003a).

As the milk flow rate from a bottle increases, the rate of swallowing must also increase, which contributes to the interruption of ventilation. As the respiratory system in a late preterm infant can already be compromised, yet another challenge to breathing may result in further complications and difficulty breastfeeding.

## Delayed Lactogenesis II and Insufficient Milk Production

The first 14 days following delivery is the time when milk synthesis and production calibrate to a level sufficient for optimal growth of the infant. In term mothers, daily milk transfer on day 5 during breastfeeding has been measured at 415 ± 123 mL (14.03 oz ± 4.1 oz), increasing to daily milk transfer of 653 ± 154 mL (22 oz ± 5.2 oz) during the second week postpartum. Ninety-two percent of term mothers produce at least a minimum 440 mL (13.5 oz) per day by two weeks of lactation (Kent et al., 2016).

In a study of 142 mothers of preterm infants, the prevalence of delayed lactogenesis was 36%, with delayed milk expression initiation and pregnancy induced hypertension serving as major risk factors (Yu et al., 2019). In this study, milk volumes in the delayed-lactogenesis group during every 24-hour period through the first 14 days postpartum was significantly less than in the non-delayed lactogenesis group (Yu et al., 2019). Many factors, however, conspire to challenge sufficient milk production in a mother of a late preterm infant (Briere et al., 2015; Meier et al., 2007; Walker, 2008) (Table 5).

**Table 5.** Challenges to milk production in late preterm mothers

| Challenge to milk production | Effect on milk production |
|---|---|
| Separation at birth | Prevents skin-to-skin contact, eliminates direct infant stimulation of the breast, requires mother to artificially initiate lactation by hand expression and/or pumping. |
| Weak suction of infant | Infant suck may be inadequate to properly stimulate milk production. |
| Uncoordinated suck, swallow, breathe process | Infant may fail to adequately stimulate milk production. |
| Fatigue prior to completing a feeding | Infant may not adequately drain the breast, giving false signals of milk volume required to be synthesized. |
| Inability to regulate sleep/ wake cycles; baby sleepy or falling asleep at the breast | Infant may have inadequate number of feedings per 24 hours serving to downregulate milk production. |
| Reliance on breast pump for initiating and maintaining milk production | A pump may not be efficient in initiating and maintaining milk production; mother may not pump sufficient number of times. |
| Delayed lactogenesis II | Delayed LG II may be complicated by cesarean delivery, pregnancy-induced hypertension, high maternal BMI, or maternal diabetes. Delayed LG II adversely affects interplay between the systemic lactation hormones and autocrine control of lactation at the level of the individual breast through the feedback inhibitor of lactation mechanism. Ineffective milk removal over several days downregulates milk volume through both systemic and local responses. |

| Stress (long difficult labor, posttraumatic stress, stress to mother and infant during labor, urgent cesarean section) | Delayed onset of lactation (Dewey, 2001; Dimitraki et al., 2016; Hobbs et al, 2016). |
|---|---|
| Supplementation with a feeding bottle and artificial nipple | Sucking on an artificial nipple can weaken the strength of the suck, change the mouth conformation, extinguish the extrusion reflex, and cause the infant to prefer the artificial nipple over the maternal nipple. |

## Maternal Conditions

Lactogenesis II can be delayed in the presence of maternal diabetes (DeBortoli & Amir, 2016). Earlier studies showed that the onset of lactogenesis II in women with insulin dependent diabetes mellitus could be delayed between 15 and 28 hours (Arthur et al., 1989; Hartmann & Cregan, 2001; Neubauer et al., 1993). Not all women with gestational diabetes experience delayed lactogenesis, but women with gestational diabetes who are treated with insulin for the condition are at a significantly higher risk for delayed lactogenesis (Matias et al., 2014).

Significantly greater odds of a history of diabetes has been observed in women with a low milk supply. Riddle and Nommsen-Rivers (2016) reported that women diagnosed with low milk supply were significantly more likely to have had diabetes in pregnancy compared with women with latch or nipple problems and, more generally, compared with women with any other lactation difficulty. Healthy insulin dynamics seems an important contributor to the timely onset of lactogenesis II and sufficient milk production.

Women with a high pre-pregnancy body mass index (BMI) have a higher rate of delayed lactogenesis than women with a low BMI (Turcksin et al., 2014). Excessive gestational weight gain also predisposes women to delayed lactogenesis (Preusting et al., 2017). The mean onset of lactogenesis in this study for women with a BMI >30 was 85.2 hours postpartum, with the cutoff for the definition of delayed lactogenesis II being 72 hours. Some studies with small samples have found that overweight and obese women have been reported to experience a decrease in the prolactin response to suckling (Babendure et al., 2015; Rasmussen & Kjolhede, 2004), disrupting an important hormonal influence on milk synthesis. Obesity is known to increase insulin resistance that may delay the time it takes to reach an insulin concentration sufficient enough for the onset of lactation. Insulin has been shown to be necessary for secretory activation of the breasts and mature milk production (Nommsen-Rivers, 2016).

# Parental Perceptions and Experiences of Breastfeeding a Late Preterm Infant

Some parents may not comprehend the difference between a late preterm and term newborn. They may have formed the impression that even though the baby was a little early, it didn't mean that they should expect much difference in the behavior and skills of their newborn compared with a full-term infant. When clinicians have not provided anticipatory guidance regarding what to expect, many of the challenges, such as feeding, will come as a surprise to parents. The "normalization" of late preterm infants could predispose parents to stress and distress when they encounter the reality of dealing with the manifestations of late preterm immaturity (Premji et al., 2017).

If discharged soon after birth, parents bear the further responsibility of monitoring for jaundice, weight loss, dehydration, and hypoglycemia, and require education regarding these potential conditions and how to prevent them. Parents may not be prepared for the inconsistent, disorganized, and variable behaviors surrounding

**Box 1.** Breastfeeding difficulties identified by mothers

## Latch difficulties
- Small mouth that could not surround the nipple
- Sliding on and off the breast
- Shallow latch
- Disorganized feeding behavior

## Frequent feedings
- Lack of consistent feedings with every feeding being different
- Stress and distress at the breast
- Weak suck
- Sleepy at the breast/falling asleep before feeding is finished
- Infant fatigue
- Confusing infant fatigue at breast with satiation
- Gagging and choking on both breast and bottle
- Prolonged feedings
- Exhaustion of both mother and baby during frustrating feeds
- Not knowing if baby was getting enough at each feeding
- Excessive time investment in feeding

## Healthcare provider lack of knowledge
- Pushing supplementation with formula
- Contradictory information and interventions
- Lack of support
- No anticipatory guidance
- Lack of consistent breastfeeding plan

breastfeeding. Premji et al. (2017) noted in their study that mothers failed to recognize signs of feeding distress in their infant (tongue thrusting, milk pooling or dribbling, splayed fingers, and eyes widening), and labelled them as typical feeding behaviors. Many mothers also did not perform interventions to manage the feeding distress.

Late preterm infants with limited breastfeeding skills and reduced breastfeeding efficiency and who are presented with one or more perinatal challenge are at high risk for slow or no weight gain or weight loss, dehydration, hypoglycemia, hyperbilirubinemia, formula supplementation, and abandonment of breastfeeding. Mothers of late preterm babies want to breastfeed their infants but have identified difficulties with feeding as a significant issue in caring for their newborn(Box 1.) (Dosani et al., 2017).

The frustrating nature of breastfeeding late preterm infants can lead to formula supplementation with bottles and a downward spiral to abandonment of breastfeeding. With the continued frustrations and apparent lack of progress with feeding difficulties, some mothers wait until breastfeeding is severely threatened before seeking reliable breastfeeding support. They often turn to the Internet, social media, friends, and healthcare providers who lack the expertise to provide effective interventions (Demirci et al., 2015). Many mothers of late preterm infants will need to express their milk in addition to providing frequent feeds at the breast. This compounds time investment, can increase maternal fatigue, and add more stress to an already stressful situation.

Consistent feeding plans are vital with close follow-up until the infant is successfully breastfeeding. Failure to latch and breastfeed successfully may lead some mothers to exclusively pump their milk in order to assure that their infant receives breastmilk for as long as possible. Guidelines will need to be provided for these mothers regarding pump selection, pumping, handling, storing, and using the pumped milk, as well as interventions if problems are encountered, such as insufficient milk production. Small, achievable goals are helpful, as sometimes breastfeeding late preterm infants is a "waiting game," where infant maturation towards term dates brings partial or total relief to the situation. Clinicians will need to monitor these mother/baby dyads more closely in the hospital and in the community following discharge, making sure that parents have been informed and prepared for the challenges that await.

# SECTION TWO

# Breastfeeding Management Guidelines

Several protocols and practice guidelines have been published for both the overall care of late preterm infants, as well as specifically for breast-feeding the late preterm infant. These can serve as starting points for evidence-based recommendations and interventions (Table 6).

**Table 6.** Protocols and guidelines for the care and breastfeeding of late preterm infants

| Protocol/guideline | Source | Comments |
|---|---|---|
| *Multidisciplinary guidelines for the care of late preterm infants* (Phillips et al., 2013) | National Perinatal Association http://www.nationalperinatal.org/latepreterm | Includes recommendations for the healthcare team, as well as recommended family education suggestions |
| Care and management of the late preterm infant | California Perinatal Quality Care Collaborative https://www.cpqcc.org/content/care-and-management-late-preterm-infant-0 | Comprehensive toolkit |
| Late-preterm infants: A population at risk (Engle et al., 2007) | American Academy of Pediatrics https://pediatrics.aappublications.org/content/120/6/1390 | Policy was reaffirmed June 2018 |
| *ABM Clinical Protocol #10: Breastfeeding the late preterm and early term infants* (Boies & Vaucher, 2016) | Academy of Breastfeeding Medicine https://abm.memberclicks.net/assets/DOCUMENTS/PROTOCOLS/10-breastfeeding-the-late-pre-term-infant-protocol-english.pdf | Includes breastfeeding recommendations for both late preterm and early term infants |

| Protocol/guideline | Source | Comments |
|---|---|---|
| SPIN: Supporting Premature Infant Nutrition | UC San Diego SPIN Program https://health.ucsd.edu/ SPECIALTIES/OBGYN/ MATERNITY/NEWBORN/ NICU/SPIN/Pages/default.aspx | Comprehensive resource with materials for both clinicians and parents |
| *Assessment and care of the late preterm infant* (2nd edition) | Association of Women's Health, Obstetric and Neonatal Nurses https://www.awhonn. org/store/ViewProduct. aspx?id=9356391 | Addresses a broad range of risks associated with late preterm birth |

Late preterm infants are at a disadvantage in terms of feeding skills (Box 2).

**Box 2.** Limitations on Feeding Skills of Late Preterm Infants

### Low energy stores and high energy demands

- Limited amounts of subcutaneous fat and brown fat to draw upon for energy.

### Sleepy with fewer and shorter awake periods

- Presents fewer feeding cues that may be more difficult to recognize.

### Tire easily when feeding

- Exhibit decreased endurance and may not be able to demonstrate enough stamina to transfer adequate amounts of colostrum or milk at a feeding.

### Low muscle tone

- May result in inability to create high enough vacuum levels to remove milk from the breast. Rapid decrease in tone during a feeding, a poor seal on the breast, and difficulty maintaining the nipple in the oral cavity with a maintenance vacuum of about -60 mmHg compromises milk intake. Improved muscle tone may be gained with the muscle conditioning provided by the act of feeding at the breast.

## Weak suck

- Vacuum generation is central to breastmilk removal. Late preterm infants have difficulty maintaining a sustained negative pressure. Infants need to generate a vacuum of approximately $-145 \pm 58$ mm Hg to optimize milk flow from the breast (Geddes et al., 2008). Low vacuum generation or inability to modify sucking dynamics to adapt to changes in milk flow following the conclusion of a milk-ejection reflex can result in insufficient milk transfer (Cannon et al., 2016).

- Even though they may latch better, preterm infants have been shown to generate a weaker intra-oral vacuum when sucking over a nipple shield compared to full-term infants (Geddes et al., 2017).

## Altered sucking patterns

- Sucking patterns differ from a full-term infant, as preterm infants tend to exhibit more single sucks rather than performing sucking bursts of 10 or more sucks, further reducing milk intake (Geddes et al., 2017).

## Inconsistent feeding patterns

- Infant decreased responsiveness, feed-to-feed variation in milk transfer, and lack of consistent feeding and satiety cues results in day-to-day oscillation in feeding effectiveness (Demirci et al., 2015).

- The creation of a breastfeeding plan of care for late preterm infants is predicated by their vulnerabilities and challenges (Boies & Vaucher, 2016). Breastfeeding management options for this population are often extrapolated from those used with either full-term infants or with infants less than 34 weeks of gestation, neither of which may be completely appropriate for the unique needs of late preterm infants. Not all interventions have been well researched, but all protocols should strive to prevent adverse outcomes, establish an abundant maternal milk supply, assure adequate infant intake, and consider the emotional toll taken on the parents of these babies.

# Getting Started with Breastfeeding

## Skin-to-Skin Care

Avoiding early separation and keeping infants skin to skin with their mothers enhances breastfeeding initiation and extends breastfeeding duration (Moore et al., 2016). If the infant has experienced a vaginal birth and is stable, this is the first step in a breastfeeding plan. Some hospitals provide skin-to-skin care in the operating room following a cesarean delivery, resulting in better outcomes and fewer transfers to the neonatal intensive care unit (NICU) (Schneider et al., 2017). Skin to skin in the operating room has shown a statistically positive association with exclusive breastfeeding rates on discharge and at 3 and 6 months (Guala et al., 2017).

Skin-to-skin is an important strategy in the prevention of hypothermia, hypoglycemia, toxic stress, crying, and the excessive or unnecessary burning of calories. It provides the infant with a time and place to engage in the 9 stages of instinctive behavior that allow the infant to perform the behavior patterns practiced in utero as a "survival mechanism" (Widstrom et al., 2020) (Table 7).

Infants who undergo the nine stages during skin-to-skin care may be more likely to successfully and exclusively breastfeed (Crenshaw et al., 2012). Disruption of this behavior pattern should be avoided if possible, to facilitate a counter mechanism to the breastfeeding challenges that late preterm infants already face.

**Table 7.** Widstrom's nine stages of instinctual behavior and the parallel fetal movements (Widstrom et al., 2011; Widstrom et al., 2020).

| Widstrom Stage | Emergence | Fetal Behavior Pattern | Emergence |
|---|---|---|---|
| 1. The birth cry | At birth; Moro reflex | Startle reflex | Week 9 to 10 |
| 2. Relaxation | After birth cry as a pause in activity | | |
| 3. Awakening- increase in small body movements | 2.5 minutes following birth | Whole slow body movements | Week 9 to 10 |
| 4. Activity- larger body movements | 8 minutes following birth | Generalized body movements | Week 9+ to 10+ |
| 5. Rest- periodically between activity periods | Throughout first hour following birth | Rest periods between active movements | |
| 6. Crawling-step reflex initiated as a crawling motion | 36 minutes following birth | Occasional coordinated leg movements and "kicking" | Week 11 |
| 7. Familiarization- brushes and licks areola, mouthing movements over nipple | 43 minutes following birth | Head and hand movements more coordinated | Week 11+ |
| 8. Suckling-has latched to nipple and begins sucking | 62 minutes following birth | Sucking and swallowing movements; swallows amniotic fluid | Week 12+ |
| 9. Sleeping- movements diminish as newborn closes eyes into deeper sleep | 90 minutes following birth | Sleep patterns emerge | Week 30+ |

Infants from a medicated labor progress through the nine stages but certain medications, like fentanyl, may suppress the newborn's sucking behavior. If the mother and newborn were unable to experience the first hours together, or the infant did not latch and suck before falling asleep, then providing as much skin-to-skin contact as possible during the hospital stay becomes very important. There is concern regarding the occurrence of Sudden Unexpected Postnatal Collapse (SUPC), and the potential association with skin-to-skin contact and respiratory distress (to which the late preterm infant may be prone). Close monitoring of skin-to-skin by hospital staff is important during the early time following birth.

Parents should be educated regarding safe positioning by discussion with their nurse and the use of a tool such as a card, handout, or poster (Ludington-Hoe & Morgan, 2014) (Figure 4). Safe positioning instructions to parents can include the following:

- Set the bed at about a 35-degree angle so she is elevated, not flat nor completely upright

- Baby is belly down, chest to chest

- Baby's head should be turned to the side so you can see the face

- The head should be in a "sniffing" position; slightly looking up

- Shoulders are flat against mom

- Nose and mouth are not covered

- Baby's back is covered with a light blanket

- Mothers should give their babies their full attention without distractions like smartphones

- Someone is watching the mother and baby

- If the mother is sleepy, place baby on his/her back in a bassinet or the in the arms of another alert caregiver

**Figure 4.** Safe positioning for skin-to-skin care.
Source: Ken Tackett. Blanket is removed so baby's position is visible.

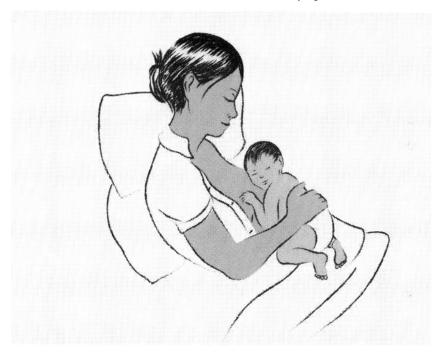

## Positioning

The first hour after birth is a physiologically sensitive or critical period. The infant experiences an increased sensitivity to the odor of colostrum while the very high levels of catecholamines strengthen memory and learning (Widstrom et al., 2019). Late preterm infants may benefit from initially breastfeeding when the mother is in a semi-reclining or laid-back position.

The dorsal or prone positioning of the infant releases the primitive neonatal reflexes that are associated with establishing successful breastfeeding. These reflexes include, but are not limited to, hand to mouth, mouth gape, tongue dart, head bob, rooting, palmar grasp, crawl, suck, jaw jerk, swallow head lift, and hand reflex. Significantly more primitive neonatal reflexes have been observed as stimulants to successful breastfeeding when mothers were in a semi-reclined position as compared to mothers who were sitting upright or side-lying (Colson et al., 2008) (Figure 5).

**Figure 5.** Laid-back positioning of newborns.
Photo courtesy of Lucia Jenkins, RN, IBCLC, RLC.

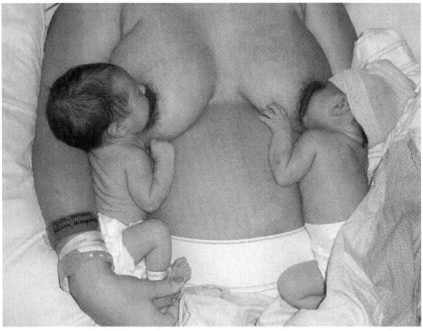

The dorsal or prone position of the infant can help improve infant oxygenation and facilitate eye contact of mother and infant, which may increase maternal oxytocin pulsatility (Colson, 2014). The laid-back position keeps both the infant and mother from having to expend energy fighting the effects of gravity on positioning. Rather than the head and back of the infant being pulled away from the breast by gravity, as in upright positions, prone positioning uses gravity to keep mother and baby connected, and allows the infant chin and tongue to move down and forward, increasing the likelihood of a successful latch.

Modifications to positioning are always in order if the mother has had a cesarean delivery or has large or pendulous breasts that would make laid-back positioning awkward. Cross cradle or clutch positions are also options. The mother's breast should not rest on the baby's chest in the clutch position. Some late preterm infants may demonstrate respiratory instability in certain positions. They are more prone to positional apnea due to airway obstruction, as they lack postural control in their neck. The traditional cradle hold may not be suitable for late preterm infants, as the neck can become so flexed that the airway is blocked, and full rib cage expansion is impeded.

## Hypotonia and Immature Feeding Skills

Some late preterm infants can effectively latch, suck, and swallow colostrum and milk, especially with jaw support. Others may tire quickly, be unable to sustain nutritive sucking, or they lack the strength to draw the nipple/areola into the mouth and generate the necessary vacuum to keep it there. Hypotonia of the oral musculature used to grasp the nipple, generate the vacuum necessary to draw the nipple/areola into the mouth, hold it there, and sustain nutritive sucking can contribute to uncoordinated and ineffective milk transfer.

The physiologic maturity necessary to establish effective suck/swallow/breathe coordination manifests at the time that late preterm infants are born, so the challenge to breastfeeding is not surprising. Infants' intraoral vacuum pressure varies, which changes over the duration of a single feeding (Alatalo et al., 2020). Vacuum levels that drop too low cause the infant to lose the latch, continuously have to re-latch, and diminish the volume of colostrum and milk that can be extracted from the breast.

Sucking patterns are often erratic and immature. Nyqvist et al. (2001) used surface electromyography in a study of sucking patterns during breastfeeding in 26 infants aged 32 to 37 weeks. The time spent sucking ranged from 10% and 60% of a feeding, while mouthing movements other than sucking ranged from 2% to 35% of the feeding. Pauses ranged from 12% to 67%.

Late preterm infants have been shown to have blunted rooting responses, no or shallow latch, short latch duration, shorter sucking bursts, occasional swallowing rather than repeated swallowing, and short feeding durations (Pike et al., 2017). Pike et al. (2017) also showed that more infants exhibited the most mature behavior for each feeding characteristic when the environment was quiet rather than noisy and disturbing. Late preterm infants typically consume breastmilk in small volumes during the first few days of life but may be unable to consume higher volumes of breastmilk needed for sufficient growth following hospital discharge (Ludwig, 2007).

Maturation may eventually improve hypotonia and immature feeding skills, but mothers need specific and clear feeding plans during this time. Frequent opportunities to suckle at the breast, even if it is non-nutritive sucking, can improve the transition to effective breastfeeding. Suck training is a general term applied to exercises that are designed to improve different aspects of sucking (Marmet & Shell, 1984).

There are no standardized suck-improvement techniques but a common one, if the infant tolerates it, is the finger tug, which is designed to improve muscle strength. This involves allowing the infant to draw a clean index finger into the mouth, begin sucking, and then slightly withdrawing the finger allowing the infant to suck it back in. Gentle stroking or massage of the lips, cheeks, and jaw may prime the infant for sucking motions. Based on each infant's response and situation, oral-strengthening exercises may be recommended by therapists (speech and language, occupational, physical) trained in infant oral motor therapy.

# Latching and Latch Assistance

The latch is probably the most important moment and movement in the breastfeeding process. When brushed with the nipple/areola or after sucking stimulation, if needed, the infant's open mouth grasps the nipple, pulling it and part of the areola deeply into the mouth. The nipple/areola complex needs to be drawn deep enough into the mouth for effective sucking, generally at or more often to right before the junction of the hard and soft palate (Jacobs et al., 2007). The infant's mouth should open wide, up to a 160° angle (Figure 6).

**Figure 6.** Wide open mouth with optimal mouth opening angle. From Wilson-Clay & Hoover, 2002.

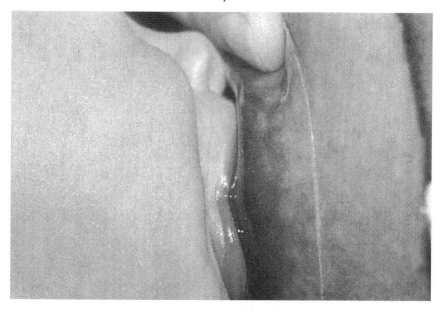

The neck may be slightly extended to assure that the mandible can lower to appropriately open the mouth. Too much flexion in the neck with distortion of the cervical vertebrae can impinge on the proper movement of the hyoid bone, which has connections involved in sucking, swallowing, and breathing. The infant's head should not be pushed or forced into the breast, as it may disturb placement of the tongue, encouraging it to elevate rather than cup and move down and forward.

Poor attachment to the breast that leaves the nipple in the anterior portion of the mouth can contribute to maternal sore nipples, obstructed milk flow, infant weight loss, jaundice, and low milk supply. A deep latch facilitates uniform drainage of all the mammary lobes. Mizuno and colleagues (2008) found that the degree of emptying of each mammary lobe differed by the depth of the latch. A deep latch was defined as the nipple plus 0.7 to 1.3 cm of the areola drawn into the infant's mouth and the angle of the open mouth greater than 130 degrees. If the depth of attachment was shallow, milk was secreted unevenly from different mammary lobes, potentially predisposing the breast to plugged ducts and mastitis. If a lobe is poorly drained over time, less milk will be synthesized in that lobe, and milk production may decrease.

Some infants may need assistance in opening their mouth wide enough to create an effective latch. Mothers or a helper can **gently** exert downward pressure on the chin to open the mouth and turn out the lower lip (Wolf & Glass, 1992) (Figure 7).

If the infant has diminished muscle tone, providing extra jaw support from the Dancer hand position may help stabilize the jaw such that the infant does not keep slipping off of the nipple or does not bite or clench the jaw to keep from sliding off the breast (Danner & Cerutti, 1984) (Figure 8).

**Figure 7.** Gently opening the infant's mouth to facilitate latch.
Photo courtesy of Marsha Walker.

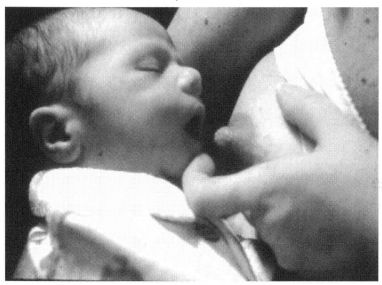

**Figure 8.** Dancer hand position. From Wilson-Clay & Hoover, 2002.

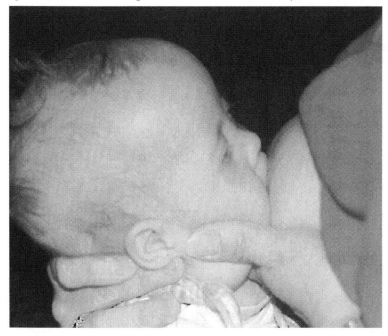

If the infant latches, but smacking sounds can be heard, this may mean that the infant's tongue is losing contact with the nipple/areola as the jaw drops down too far. Sublingual support may be useful to keep the tongue in contact with the breast. Sublingual support is done when the mother slips her index finger directly behind and under the tip of the chin where the tongue attaches. This limits the downward movement of the jaw so that suction is not lost each time the jaw drops.

An edematous areola may complicate latch attempts. While the nipple may appear to be flat, it can be enveloped by the swollen areolar tissue, making it more difficult for the infant to draw in the excess tissue. Placing a vacuum pump on swollen tissue to evert the nipple may exacerbate the problem. If the areola is engorged, areolar compression (Miller & Riordan, 2004) or reverse pressure softening (Cotterman, 2004) can displace fluid in the areola for an easier latch. This involves the mother pressing her fingers around the areola to make indentations or pits that serve to temporarily displace fluid and expose the nipple (Figure 9).

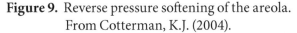

**Figure 9.**  Reverse pressure softening of the areola.
From Cotterman, K.J. (2004).

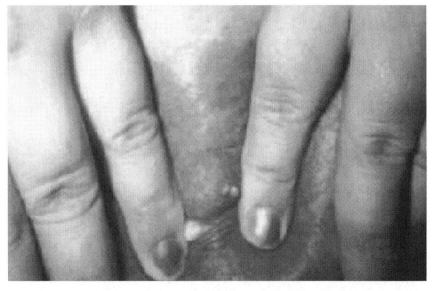

If the nipple is flat (not enveloped by an edematous areola) and compromising the latch, consider using a modified syringe to evert the nipple (Kesaree et al., 1993). A 10 mL syringe (or larger to accommodate a larger nipple) is modified by cutting ¼" above where the needle attaches, removing the plunger, and inserting it into the cut end (Figure 10). Prior to a feeding, the smooth end is placed over the nipple and the mother pulls back gently on the plunger for 30 seconds. While this syringe modification is not an FDA approved device, there are a number of commercial devices on the market used to evert flat nipples that may be approved for this use. Some mothers find that using a breast pump prior to feedings can help.

**Figure 10.** Modified syringe to evert a flat nipple. (From Kesaree et al., 1993).

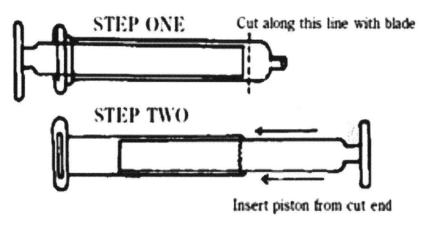

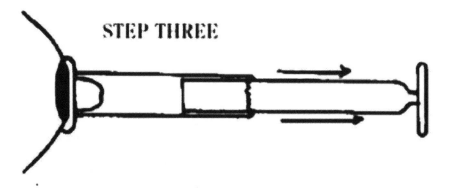

If the infant remains unable to effectively latch, then latch incentives may help. One technique for providing a latch incentive is for the clinician to use a milk-filled dropper placed in the side of the infant's mouth as the baby moves to latch. As the infant's mouth envelopes, the nipple/areola, a drop or two of milk can be placed on the tongue to encourage a swallow followed by a nutritive suck (Figure 11).

**Figure 11.** A milk incentive causes the infant to swallow and follow with a nutritive suck. Photo courtesy of Marsha Walker.

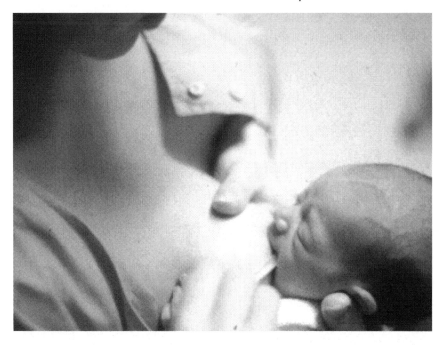

Some infants, especially when hungry, demonstrate a deteriorating behavioral pattern at the breast with rapid side-to-side head movements or arching away from the breast. An intervention to help this infant latch is for the clinician to use a milk-filled dropper and as the mother guides the baby to the breast, touch the midline of the upper lip with the tip of the dropper to stop the movement as the baby orients to this touch. The dropper tip remains on the upper lip and is used to guide the infant forward onto the breast. As the baby latches, a drop or two of milk can be placed in the mouth to encourage a swallow followed by a nutritive suck (Figure 12).

**Figure 12.** Dropper assisted latch stops rapid
side-to-side head movements. Photo courtesy of Marsha Walker.

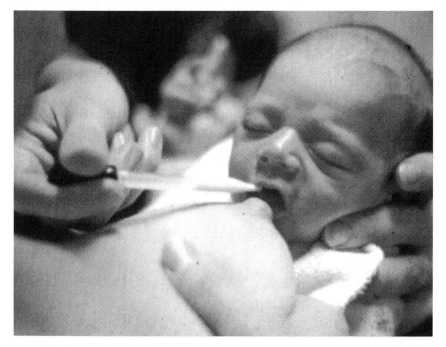

A tube feeding device or periodontal syringe can also be used as a latch incentive with the tubing or syringe tip placed in the corner of the infant's mouth during the latch sequence. Once the infant has latched, assistance may be needed to help sustain the sucking. Alternate massage/breast compressions (Figure 13) may be helpful to keep the infant latched and interested, especially during the pauses between sucking bursts. The mother massages and compresses the breast either during the pause or during the suck, whichever works best. This helps improve the pressure gradient between breast and mouth, reducing the effort necessary to withdraw milk.

The infant generally starts sucking again after the breast has been compressed, helping to improve milk transfer and increase the volume of colostrum/milk consumed. Mothers should make sure that all quadrants of each breast are massaged and compressed to prevent milk stasis and a downregulation of milk production from lack of lobular drainage.

**Figure 13.** Breast compressions alternating with sucking bursts. From *Dr. Jack Newman's Visual Guide to Breastfeeding,* Kernerman & Newman, 2007.

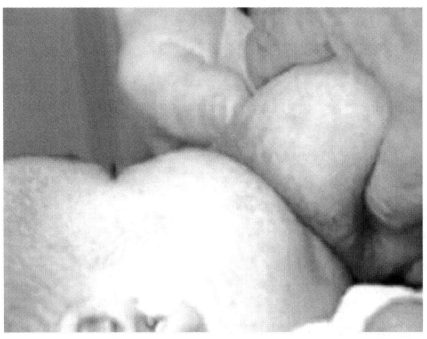

If other latch-assist techniques fail to improve the infant's latch, use of an ultrathin silicone nipple shield might be helpful to initiate latch and keep the infant from repeatedly losing contact with the nipple or slipping off the breast, necessitating multiple attempts to re-latch. Nipple shields have been used with preterm infants to compensate for weak intraoral vacuum and as a temporary device to encourage successful latching to the breast until vacuum pressures increase to that of full-term infants (Meier et al., 2007). However, some researchers found that using a nipple shield with late preterm infants was associated with lower rates breastfeeding exclusively during the first week at home or at 1 month and feeding less than 10 times per day (Jonsdottir et al., 2020).

Geddes et al. (2017) measured intraoral vacuum in preterm infants and showed that the vacuum generated was lower when a nipple shield was used compared to when no nipple shield was in place. The authors speculated that different size shields might position the nipple differently in the oral cavity. If the tip of the shield was positioned too close to the junction of the hard and soft palate, it might only allow a small milk bolus to be removed or discourage sucking. If the shield placed the nipple too far away from the hard and soft palate junction in the anterior portion of the mouth, then the amount of vacuum applied to the shield and nipple might compromise the volume of milk that could be removed from the breast.

Rather than the immediate use of a nipple shield, it may be prudent to allow the infant to imprint on the maternal nipple first, perhaps during the first 12 to 24 hours following delivery (supplementing if needed) (Walker, 2016). Imprinting in infants has been described as a stage in neurodevelopment whereby the infant recognizes the mother through oral tactile memory (Mobbs et al., 2016). Introduction of a nipple shield with its stiff teat and different size and texture than the maternal nipple could act as a super stimulus, provoking a preference for the artificial nipple over the real thing. The newborn period is a critical developmental window of time where the brain and nervous system are especially sensitive to certain environmental stimuli. If an infant does not experience an appropriate stimulus (such as the maternal nipple) during this period, it might make it more difficult to learn the appropriate sucking skills later-on.

Nipple shields come in different sizes so matching the size to both the maternal nipple and the infant's mouth may take some trial and error. Too small a shield may pinch or result in sore nipples while too large a shield may prohibit the infant from properly latching onto it. Some mothers may need a different size shield for each breast.

To help the shield adhere better to the breast, the shield can be moistened with warm water and turned almost inside out when applying it to the nipple (Figure 14).

**Figure 14.** Applying a nipple shield. Photo courtesy of Marsha Walker.

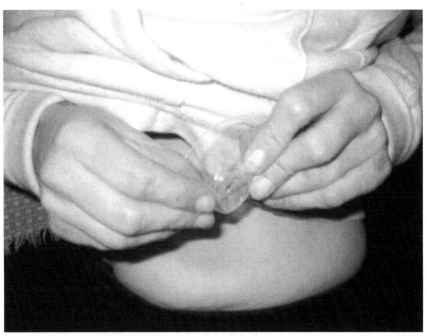

This helps the shield stay in place better and places the nipple as far into the nipple tunnel as possible. The mother can hand express some colostrum/milk into the shield teat to make it immediately available to any amount of sucking, or the clinician can pre-fill the shield teat using a periodontal syringe, injecting milk through one of the teat openings after the shield is in place on the breast.

Once the nipple has been drawn into the shield, a vacuum in the semi-rigid teat assures that the nipple stays elongated and lowers the workload on the baby of having to constantly draw the nipple/areola back into the mouth. A few drops of colostrum or milk can be placed on the tip of the shield to encourage latch on. The infant should be checked to make sure that the lips and gums completely cover the shield teat (Figure 6) and that the baby is not just gumming or chewing on the tip of the shield.

Mothers should check that all areas of each breast are adequately drained while using a shield. An older study reported a 12% rate of mastitis in mothers who still used a shield at 3 months postpartum (Nicholson, 1993). A study looking at the contributors to mastitis showed that mothers who used nipple shields had a two-fold increased risk of developing mastitis compared to women who did not use a shield (Cullinane et al., 2015).

Clinicians may wish to advise mothers to periodically massage and compress each quadrant of each breast during feedings to reduce the chance of leaving pockets of retained milk. If the infant cannot transfer sufficient milk with the shield in place, and is unable to latch without it, a tube from a tube-feeding device can be placed under or on top of the shield to deliver pumped milk supplements.

As the infant's sucking improves, latch can be tried without the shield, or it can be removed partway through a feeding as weaning from the shield progresses. Shields should be washed in hot soapy water, rinsed well, and air dried between feedings. There are no generally agreed-upon or professionally peer-reviewed protocols, policies, or algorithms for nipple shield use (Eglash et al., 2010), but suggested nipple shield guidelines can be found in Table 8.

Table 8. Suggested guidelines for nipple shield use.

| Action | Rationale |
|---|---|
| Recommend a nipple shield if the clinical situation warrants it. | Not all special situations require a shield. Shield use may preserve breastfeeding in selected situations. |
| If a nipple shield is required during the initial hospital stay, allow the infant to feed or attempt to feed at the breast at least once or twice before introducing a shield. | Allow the infant to imprint on the maternal nipple first. Shield use during the hospital stay may help prevent excessive weight loss prior to discharge and avoid the use of supplemental bottles |
| Recommend the right size and shaped shield as the situation warrants. Start with a medium size shield, use a larger one if the shield pinches, if the maternal nipple is large, or if there is pain. Use the smallest shield that gives the best results. A cut out shield may be prudent for early use to allow olfaction to guide the infant to the breast. A cherry shaped shield may be helpful if the infant has difficulty latching to the conical shield. | Clinicians may need to try a number of different shields in order to secure the best fit and outcome. |
| Advise the mother to warm the shield under hot water prior to application, turn it almost inside out to apply, hand express colostrum or milk into the teat or use a periodontal syringe to preload the teat with milk. | Warming helps the shield adhere better and promotes milk ejection. Proper application allows the maternal nipple to be drawn into the shield's teat. Milk in the teat provides immediate availability so that infants with a weak suck do not become fatigued while initiating milk flow. |
| Have the mother massage and compress the breast periodically during the feeding. | This may prevent milk stasis, plugged ducts, and mastitis. |
| Pump following feedings if milk production is low or the risk for a compromised milk supply is high. | Milk production must be monitored to assure an abundant supply and that the shield is not contributing to milk supply reduction. |

| Action | Rationale |
|---|---|
| Check to make sure that the shield is properly applied, that the infant is latched appropriately and is transferring milk, and that the mother knows how to clean the shield. Recommend frequent weight checks | Shield use should not reinforce improper latching. Milk transfer monitoring is important to assure proper infant weight gain and an abundant milk supply. |
| Recommend that the mother make an appointment with an IBCLC for continued follow-up. Walker, M. (2016). | Professional follow-up is required for assessing and monitoring any ongoing problems or issues that necessitated shield use. |

## The Latchable State

Because more than one-third of the brain volume at term is acquired during the last 6 to 8 weeks of gestation, late preterm infants are at a disadvantage in responding to stimuli and regulating internal processes. Karl (2004) described behavioral breastfeeding difficulties on a continuum, from the under-aroused sleepy baby, through the quiet alert state (optimal for feeding) to the over-aroused, fussy reluctant nurser. For infants unable to manage their state well enough to latch, skin-to-skin care can be initiated to modulate infant state for the under-aroused, over-aroused, or shut-down infant. Handouts can be provided to parents, and posters can be displayed in hospital birthing areas encouraging parents and clinicians to keep infants in skin-to-skin contact with their mothers (Figures 15 & 16).

**Figure 15.** Handout/poster encouraging mothers to keep
their infant skin-to-skin during the hospital stay.
From the Massachusetts Breastfeeding Coalition, www.massbfc.org.

# Get to know your baby
## and let your baby know you

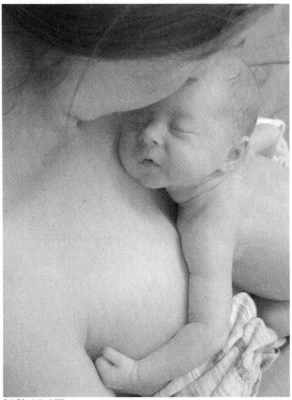

**Babies who room-in and are skin-to-skin get to:**

*For a great start, nurse your baby in the
first hour of life and plan on rooming-in.*

♥ smell you
♥ hear you
♥ feel you
♥ nurse from you
♥ stay warm
♥ be calmed and
   loved by you

FIRST HUG

Photo © Pascale Wowak 2006

© Massachusetts Breastfeeding Coalition | www.massbfc.org | Design inspired by staff at Rush-Copley Medical Center, Aurora, IL.

**Figure 16.** Handout/poster encouraging skin-to-skin
care beyond the hospital stay.
From the Massachusetts Breastfeeding Coalition, www.massbfc.org.

# It's my birthday,
*give me a hug!*

## Skin-to-Skin Contact for You and Your Baby

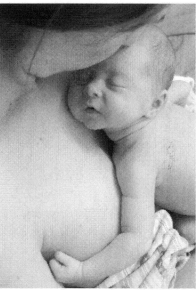

Photo © 2005 Pascale Wowak

### What's "Skin-to-Skin"?

Skin-to-skin means your baby is placed belly-down, directly on your chest, right after she is born. Your care provider dries her off, puts on a hat, and covers her with a warm blanket, and gets her settled on your chest. The first hours of snuggling skin-to-skin let you and your baby get to know each other. They also have important health benefits. If she needs to meet the pediatricians first, or if you deliver by c-section, you can unwrap her and cuddle shortly after birth. Newborns crave skin-to-skin contact, but it's sometimes overwhelming for new moms. It's ok to start slowly as you get to know your baby.

### Breastfeeding

Snuggling gives you and your baby the best start for breastfeeding. Eight different research studies have shown that skin-to-skin babies breastfeed better. They also keep nursing an average of six weeks longer. The American Academy of Pediatrics recommends that all breastfeeding babies spend time skin-to-skin right after birth. Keeping your baby skin-to-skin in his first few weeks makes it easy to know when to feed him, especially if he is a little sleepy.

### A Smooth Transition

Your chest is the best place for your baby to adjust to life in the outside world. Compared with babies who are swaddled or kept in a crib, skin-to-skin babies stay warmer and calmer, cry less, and have better blood sugars.

### Bonding

Skin-to-skin cuddling may affect how you relate with your baby. Researchers have watched mothers and infants in the first few days after birth, and they noticed that skin-to-skin moms touch and cuddle their babies more. Even a year later, skin-to-skin moms snuggled more with their babies during a visit to their pediatrician.

### Skin-to-Skin Beyond the Delivery Room

Keep cuddling skin-to-skin after you leave the hospital– your baby will stay warm and comfortable on your chest, and the benefits for bonding, soothing, and breastfeeding likely continue well after birth. Skin-to-skin can help keep your baby interested in nursing if he's sleepy. Dads can snuggle, too. Fathers and mothers who hold babies skin-to-skin help keep them calm and cozy.

### About the research

Multiple studies over the past 30 years have shown the benefits of skin-to-skin contact. In all the studies described here, mothers were randomly assigned to hold their babies skin-to-skin or see them from a distance. For more information, see Anderson GC, GC. Moore, E. Hepworth, J. Bergman, N. Early skin-to-skin contact for mothers and their healthy newborn infants. [Systematic Review] *Cochrane Pregnancy and Childbirth Group Cochrane Database of Systematic Reviews.* 2, 2005.

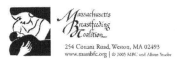

**M**assachusetts
**B**reastfeeding
**C**oalition

254 Conant Road, Weston, MA 02493
www.massbfc.org | © 2005 MBC and Alison Stuebe

Parents should be aware that stroking, rocking, talking, bright lights, loud noise, and being handed off to multiple visitors may cause the baby to shut down and be unable to latch. Infants experiencing state overload may appear to be sleeping but may be shut down in an effort to protect themselves from excessive stimulation that raised their arousal levels beyond what they can manage. Shut-down babies demonstrate tense muscle tone, furrowed eyebrows, tightly shut eyes, and a pale or flushed color. Stimulating to wake these babies further exacerbates the problem.

Mothers can be taught infant behavioral feeding cues, which are more easily recognized when the infant is skin to skin—rapid eye movements under the eyelids, sucking movements of the mouth, hand-to-mouth movements, body movements, and small sounds. Infants in a deep sleep state cannot latch but these cues are indicators of a more latchable state when the baby is more likely to feed. It is a prudent idea to limit visitors in the hospital to help minimize the dozens of interruptions that mothers experience each day during the hospital stay (Morrison et al., 2006). Some hospitals limit visiting hours and have quiet hours during the afternoon to allow mothers to rest and feed their baby.

# Assessing Feedings at the Breast

Late preterm infants' feeding competence occurs along a continuum of oral motor behaviors. The immature and disorganized sucking patterns of late preterm infants are different from the expected feeding behaviors of a full-term baby, causing clinicians and parents to alter their notion of how breastfeeding should occur. Nyqvist (2008) demonstrated that even very preterm infants (26 to 31 weeks) showed emerging competence in breastfeeding behaviors over time as they met milestones in breastfeeding capacity.

The Preterm Infant Breastfeeding Behavior Scale (PIBBS) (Table 9) may provide a useful tool to observe the emerging competence in oral motor behavior during breastfeeding over time (Nyqvist et al., 1996). Even if an infant's sucking pattern is not fully mature, the baby may still be capable of milk volume intake sufficient for adequate growth early on. Skin-to-skin care and abundant feeding practice opportunities at the breast remain important.

The PIBBS gives clinicians and parents a mechanism to track the emerging competencies and progress of the infant and help read feeding effectiveness. The items in the PIBBS are not scored, as the tool is intended for observational and tracking purposes over the continuum of skill acquisition. It can provide anticipatory guidance to the parents regarding what can be expected over time as the infant moves to a more mature feeding status.

Meeting of the milestones in the PIBBS is often an incentive to persevere with breastfeeding over the potentially many weeks it might take to achieve full breastfeeding competence. Only one study has used the PIBBS to evaluate breastfeeding competency in late preterm infants. It showed that the PIBBS was a reliable tool for clinicians and mothers that provided an objective means for evaluating feeding quality (Lober et al., 2020).

**Table 9.** The Preterm Infant Breastfeeding Bevavior Scale (PIBBS)
(From Nyqvist at al., 1996).

| Scale items | Level of competence |
|---|---|
| Rooting | • Did not root<br><br>• Showed some rooting behavior (mouth opening, tongue extension, hand-to-mouth/face movements, and head turning) |
| Areolar grasp<br>(How much of the areola is inside the baby's mouth) | • None, the mouth only touched the nipple<br><br>• Part of the nipple<br><br>• The whole nipple, not the areola<br><br>• The nipple and some of the areola |
| Sucking | • Not licking<br><br>• Licking and tasting but no sucking<br><br>• Single sucks, occasional short sucking bursts (2-9 sucks)<br><br>• Repeated (2 or more consecutive) short sucking bursts, occasional long bursts (10 sucks or more before a pause)<br><br>• Repeated long sucking bursts |
| Longest sucking bursts | • Maximum number of consecutive sucks |
| Swallowing | • Swallowing not noticed<br><br>• Occasional swallowing noticed |
| Latched to the breast | • Did not latch on at all; not felt by the mother<br><br>• Latched on for <1 minute<br><br>• Latched on for 1-15 minutes |

# Supplementation

If an infant cannot gain appropriate weight with adequate volumes of milk from direct breastfeeding, use of alternate massage/breast compressions, with a nipple shield, or with latch-assistance techniques, then supplementation may be necessary. The ideal supplement is expressed mother's own milk, or if that proves insufficient, then banked donor human milk should be used (Kellams et al., 2017). The type of supplementation has been associated with length of stay in the hospital and breastfeeding status at discharge.

Mannel and Peck (2018) found that late preterm infants who were exclusively formula-fed had longer hospital stays than exclusively breastfed infants. Breastfed infants who received *any* formula supplementation were 16% less likely to continue breastfeeding until day of discharge compared to breastfed infants who received human milk supplementation.

Breast massage has the potential for increasing the energy content in breastmilk, helping the infant ingest more calories for weight gain (Foda et al., 2004). Breast massage while pumping can also result in a higher fat content of the milk (Becker et al., 2016). If the mother has sufficient expressed breastmilk, the cream portion that rises to the top of stored milk is an option to use as a supplement.

While infant formula is a common supplement, donor human milk avoids the side effects of infant formula, such as infant gut dysbiosis, abandonment of breastfeeding, and alterations in brain growth and development. Pasteurized, donor human milk is commonly used in many neonatal intensive care units (NICU) and is increasingly being offered as a supplement in the well-baby nursery or Level I maternity units (Belfort et al., 2018).

Late preterm infants may be referred to the NICU, but many are admitted to the Level 1 or regular maternity unit. These infants should be able to benefit from an all-human milk diet too. There is a disparity in infant populations that receive banked donor milk. Some private insurers reimburse for donor human milk, as do a few state Medicaid plans. Milk banks often have a financial assistance program that will provide banked donor milk for up to one month after hospital discharge if the family is financially eligible.

There is no standard volume of supplement to deliver to late preterm infants. Anatomic stomach capacity of term infants at birth ranges from 10mL to 35mL, with an average of 20 mL gastric capacity, depending on how it is measured (Bergman, 2013). However, the amount of colostrum ingested during the first 24 hours is small, $15 \pm 11$g of colostrum (Santoro et al., 2010). The amount of colostrum seems to reflect an infant's feeding ability, as well as the physiologic volume that can comfortably fit in a stomach that is temporarily non-compliant.

The newborn stomach does not easily relax to accommodate a feeding during the early hours post birth. Over the next three days of life, the gastric tone reduces and the increased compliance allows the stomach to handle increasing volumes of milk per feeding, thus the range in suggested supplementation volumes (Zangen et al., 2001). Physiologic volumes of supplements have been suggested for healthy term infants as 2mL to 10 mL per feeding during the first 24 hours, 5mL to 15 mL from 24 to 48 hours, 15mL to 30 mL from 48 to 72 hours, and 30mL to 60 mL from 72 to 96 hours (Kellams et al., 2017). Formula-fed infants may be persuaded to consume more volume than these amounts, but this does not benefit the infants.

# Bottles

Infant feeding bottles are the most widely used feeding device for supplementing infants but come with numerous side effects. These include changes in tongue function and weakening of perioral muscles, difficulty transitioning to the breast after being bottle-fed, changes in nutritive sucking patterns, alterations in tongue positioning and lip sealing, and oxygen desaturation (Batista et al., 2019; Ferrante et al., 2006; Inoue et al., 1995; Moral et al., 2010; Thoyre & Carlson, 2003b). Artificial nipples available to the consumer have significantly different flow rates. As the milk flow increases, the infant's swallowing rate must also increase, elevating the degree of respiratory interruption and leaving fewer opportunities for breathing (al-Sayed et al., 1994).

If the infant cannot swallow fast enough, the baby may compensate by allowing milk to drool out of the mouth (Schrank et al., 1998). If the infant cannot compensate by drooling, the milk may remain in the pharynx increasing the risk for aspiration (Rommel et al., 2011). In a study that measured nipple flow rates and the variability of milk flow within the same type of nipple, researchers found that there was an extreme range of milk flow rates among artificial nipples, that the name of the nipple did not provide clear information about the flow rate, and that even among the same types and brand of nipples, the flow rates varied considerably. They recommended that in medically fragile infants starting with a truly slow flow nipple (<10 mL/minute) and one that has minimal variation among types and brands. Infants can advance to faster nipples as they tolerate the milk flow (Pados et al., 2016).

If a bottle is used, then paced feedings are important to avoid infant fatigue, bradycardia, and oxygen desaturation. Paced bottle feeding is used when infants are not able to coordinate respiration with sucking and swallowing, and engage in an immature or disorganized sucking pattern. Palmer (1993) recommends that the feeder regulate the number of sucks per sucking burst, and the duration of bursts and pauses by removing the nipple from the infant's mouth every 3 to 5 sucks, allowing a 3 to 5 second pause for breathing.

### Paced Bottle-Feeding

When the bottle is removed from the infant's mouth, the nipple rests on the midpoint of the upper lip during the breathing pauses, and remains available to allow the infant to open his mouth and draw in the nipple when ready to feed. This helps direct control of the feeding to the infant rather than having the feeder insert the nipple. Late preterm infants of younger gestational ages (34 to 35 weeks) may benefit from leaving the nipple in the baby's mouth while tipping the bottle downward to stop the flow of liquid into the mouth. During the absence of milk flow from the nipple, the infant has time to take breaths and swallow without accumulating more milk in the oral cavity (Law-Morstatt et al., 2003). Paced bottle feeding decreases the incidence of bradycardia during feedings and results in the development of more efficient sucking patterns in preterm infants (Law-Morstatt et al., 2003).

## Alternative Feeding Devices

There are several alternative feeding devices used to supplement breastfeeding infants that help avoid some of the more deleterious side effects of supplementing with a bottle and artificial nipple (Figure 17). These include spoon feeding, a feeding tube device at the breast, finger feeding with a tube-feeding device, dropper, syringe, and cup. The purposes for using such devices are to preserve the breastfeeding relationship, avoid the use of bottles and artificial nipples, and assure that infants receive adequate milk volume to support appropriate growth and development. Parents must be involved in the decision-making process for the selection of these devices.

**Figure 17.** Tube, cup, and finger feeding methods of supplementing the breastfed infant. From Stellwagen, 2007.

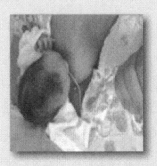

*5- or 10-mL syringe containing expressed human milk and/or formula can be attached to a 5 Fr feeding tube, the end of which should be inserted along the infant's palate after she/he has latched properly onto the breast. The syringe should be slowly pushed when the infant sucks.*

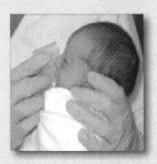

*During "cup feeding," the infant is supported in a slightly upright position. A small cup containing supplement is placed at the bottom lip to stimulate mouth opening. The cup is then tilted so that the baby can slowly sip.*

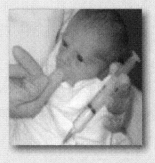

*For "finger feeding," supplement is drawn into a 5- or 1-mL syringe, which is then attached to a 5-Fr feeding tube. The end of the tube should be supported by a gloved finger when introduced into the infant's mouth. As the infant sucks on the finger, the syringe plunger can be slowly pushed.*

## Spoon Feeding

Spoon feeding a supplement (Figure 18) can be used in the early hours and days of breastfeeding when the infant requires only a small volume of supplement after each feeding attempt (Hoover, 1998). A teaspoon equals 5 mL.

**Figure 18.** Spoon feeding an infant. Sweet Sips Colostrum Spoon from https://www.sweetsipscolostrumspoons.com/

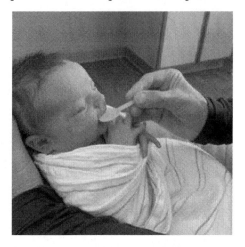

A study of preterm infants found that infants who experienced spoon feeding as a supplementation method switched to full breastfeeding sooner than a group who received bottles as a supplementation method. LATCH scores were also significantly higher among infants supplemented by spoon compared to the group supplemented with a bottle (Aytekin et al., 2014). LATCH is a breastfeeding charting system that provides a systematic method for gathering information about individual breastfeeding sessions (Jensen et al., 1994). The system assigns a numerical score, 0, 1, or 2, to five key components of breastfeeding. Each letter of the acronym LATCH denotes an area of assessment.

«L» is for how well the infant latches onto the breast. «A» is for the amount of audible swallowing noted. «T» is for the mother's nipple type. «C» is for the mother's level of comfort. «H» is for the amount of help the mother needs to hold her infant to the breast. Scores on this system can help clinicians determine where additional help is needed.

## Syringes

Syringes used to supplement infants saves time and helps feed infants with cleft lip and palate (Ize-Ilamu & Saheeb, 2011). Some clinicians prefer to use a periodontal syringe with a curved tip to deliver milk incentives at the breast or as a tool for supplementing the infant. Feeding spoons and oral syringes are inexpensive and easily available to parents following hospital discharge (Figure 19).

**Figure 19.** Colostrum spoons and oral syringes. Sweet Sips Colostrum Spoon from https://www.sweetsipscolostrumspoons.com/

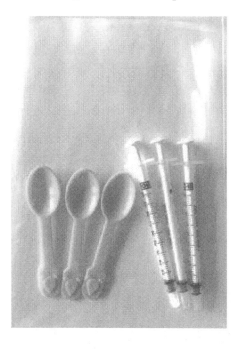

## Tube-Feeding Devices

If continued supplementation is necessary to provide larger volumes of breastmilk, tube-feeding devices might be a good option. While there is not an abundant amount of evidence for the use of tube-feeding devices, they are popular among clinicians and their use is often based on the practitioner's clinical experience (Penny et al., 2018a). Some parents may find tube-feeding devices cumbersome and time-consuming, but many appreciate using the device because they feel like they are doing something to help resolve the breastfeeding problem (Penny et al., 2018a). A simple tube-feeding device can be assembled from a 5 French feeding tube attached to a 10 mL syringe for supplementing at the breast or with finger feeding. The tubing can be taped to the breast, placed under or over a nipple shield, or held in place by a helper.

A similar device can be created from a length of butterfly tubing (with the needle removed) attached to a 20 mL or 30 mL syringe (Edgehouse & Radzyminski, 1990). Small milk boluses can be offered if needed to help the infant initiate and sustain sucking, as flow regulates suck. Commercial tube feeding systems are available for short- and long-term supplementation. The flow rate should be adjusted to either augment the flow or reduce it to avoid overwhelming a baby with immature feeding skills. If the infant is holding his breath, looking distressed, sputtering, or coughing, then the flow needs to be slowed so that a comfortable ratio of sucking to swallowing is seen and the baby inhibits breathing only when swallowing (Wolf & Glass, 2013). Care must be taken to assure a deep latch, so the infant is not simply sucking on the tubing like a straw (Guoth-Gumberger, 2006).

## Finger Feeding

Finger feeding is not well researched but can be useful for short term supplementation of larger amounts of breastmilk. You can incorporate it into a plan of care for establishing or transitioning an infant back to feeding at the breast. A tube-feeding device can be held or taped to a feeder's finger that is held pad side up as the baby is encouraged to draw the finger into his mouth. A bolus of milk is delivered to the infant after performing an effective suck. While a finger is more rigid than a breast, finger feeding encourages the infant to open the mouth wider than with an artificial nipple and draw the finger into the mouth, as the finger is not inserted as with a bottle. It would be beneficial for providers to acquire at least minimal training in the use of any alternative feeding device.

When the infant executes a correct suck with the tongue down, cupped and forward, a bolus of milk is delivered. If the infant simply bites or chews on the finger no milk is delivered. The "reward" for a correct suck shapes the desired behavior of a strong vacuum being applied with the tongue and mouth conformation that mimics sucking at the breast. Finger feeding can be used prior to a feeding to prepare the infant for attempts at breastfeeding or after a breastfeeding to deliver supplemental milk if needed. In a study of preterm infants that compared finger feeding to cup feeding, researchers found that the infants in the finger-feeding group fed more efficiently with less loss of milk than the cup-fed group (Moreira et al., 2017).

## Cup Feeding

Cup feeding has been used for decades as alternative feeding method for preterm infants. While it does not involve a transfer of learning to the breast, and does not facilitate sucking per se, cup feeding allows participation of the masseter muscles, similar to how they function in breastfeeding (Gomes et al., 2006). The masseter muscle is involved in chewing, biting, swallowing, and speech. It contributes to accurate movements of the mandible (lower jaw). Cup feeding has been shown to:

- Result in a lower incidence of oxygen desaturation episodes compared to bottle-feeding (Rocha et al., 2002),

- Establish a more stable heart rate and oxygen saturation than bottle-feeding (Penny et al., 2018b),

- Demonstrate higher rates of exclusive breastfeeding in preterm infants at discharge compared to infants who were bottle-fed (Yilmaz et al., 2014),

- Reduce the incidence of apnea and bradycardia compared with bottle-feeding (Lang et al., 1994),

- Result in significantly more mature breastfeeding behaviors compared to bottle-fed infants over 6 weeks (Abouelfettoh et al., 2008), and

- Allow the infant to control the pace and volume of the feeding with minimal risk of aspiration and minimal energy expenditure when done correctly (Dowling et al., 2002).

Cup feeding carries the possibility of spillage and a reasonable amount of milk can be lost if the technique is not done correctly. Proper technique allows the cup to be tipped only to the point where the milk touches the lower lip, with the infant licking or sipping the milk. *Milk should not be poured into the infant's mouth.* If there is significant spillage or dribbling of the milk, then supplementation may need to be done with a different alternative feeding device. Table 10 summarizes some of the strengths and limitations of many of the devices used for supplementation or for assisting the infant to feed at the breast.

**Table 10.** Advantages and Disadvantages of Alternative Feeding Devices

| Feeding Device | Advantages | Disadvantages |
|---|---|---|
| Tube feeding devices | • Allow all feedings at the breast<br><br>• Avoid artificial nipples and the potential for altering oral structure configurations<br><br>• Reinforce correct sucking patterns<br><br>• Stimulate milk production<br><br>• Deliver needed nourishment<br><br>• Allow flow rate to be adjusted to meet baby's needs<br><br>• May assist in sustaining sucking in a weakly sucking infant by providing milk flow at the breast | • Can be awkward, messy, and take time to learn<br><br>• Can be time consuming when cleaning equipment<br><br>• May be used improperly if baby sucks on the tube like a straw<br><br>• Make it difficult to feed away from home<br><br>• Can be a problem if parts break<br><br>• May be expensive for some parents |
| Finger feeding | • May help infant mimic correct oral conformation<br><br>• Requires a wide open mouth with the tongue down, cupped, and forward. Reduces tongue tip elevation<br><br>• Can be used to deliver supplement, as well as prime infant for feeding at the breast | • Can be a problem if infant displays difficulty in drawing mother's nipple/areola into the mouth because baby has become accustomed to a rigid finger<br><br>• Does not stimulate milk production |

| Feeding Device | Advantages | Disadvantages |
| --- | --- | --- |
| Syringe | • Can be used to deliver milk incentives at the breast to encourage latch<br><br>• Can be used with finger feeding to supply small amounts of milk prior to going to breast for calming purposes and suck training<br><br>• Delivers milk rewards for sucking attempts | • Often needs another person to deliver milk incentives at the breast<br><br>• Has the potential to overwhelm the infant if milk is forcefully injected into the mouth<br><br>• Is a time consuming way to feed a baby |
| Cup feeding | • Preserves function in muscles used to breastfeed<br><br>• Is easy to learn and use avoids artificial nipples<br><br>• Is a rapid way to supplement<br><br>• Is safe - reducing apnea and bradycardia seen with bottle-feeding<br><br>• Is a noninvasive alternative to gavage feeding | • Does not teach infant to feed at the breast<br><br>• May cause the loss of significant amounts of milk if infant dribbles, making intake more difficult to quantify (Dowling et al., 2002)<br><br>• Increases the risk of aspiration if milk is poured into the infant's mouth (Thorley, 1997)<br><br>• Does not increase milk production |

| Feeding Device | Advantages | Disadvantages |
|---|---|---|
| Nasogastric tube feeding in the hospital | • Assures adequate intake in infants who are unable to suck effectively, especially younger late preterm infants<br><br>• Avoids artificial nipples<br><br>• Is temporary | • Is invasive<br><br>• Does not improve milk production |
| Artificial nipples | • Are a quick and easy way to supplement<br><br>• May need to be considered if long term supplementation is necessary<br><br>• Are helpful in certain situations when specialized artificial nipples are needed | • May cause mother to abandon breastfeeding<br><br>• May overwhelm infant if nipple has a fast flow rate<br><br>• May cause apnea and bradycardia during feedings<br><br>• Alters oral conformation, tongue movement, and muscle function |

Supplementation may need to continue following discharge, sometimes until the infant reaches his due date, or even for several weeks beyond. Include information on supplementation in a discharge feeding plan. Even when adequate breastmilk is available, infants with immature breastfeeding skills may not be able to consume all of what they require until their actual due date or longer. Parents may have been given instructions on the number of ounces per day that the infant requires. Renting a digital scale can help parents measure weight changes within 1 to 2 grams. This might be appropriate post discharge when intake must be closely watched, or when determining the amount of supplement the infant needs.

Parents of late preterm infants are usually quite concerned about whether their infant is getting enough milk at each feeding, whether the baby is gaining weight, and if and how much supplement the infant may require. Because during the early days at home, late preterm infants may continue to breastfeed inefficiently, pre- and post-feed weights can validate whether the infant received sufficient intake or needs to be supplemented after a feeding, or in addition to feedings at the breast. With a suitable digital scale, parents can track weight gain over time, reducing the need for frequent trips to the infant's primary healthcare provider for simple weight checks. Supplements can be gradually decreased when they see improvement between pre- and post-feed weight checks, when adequate weight gain is seen when supplements are gradually decreased, and when increasing amounts of supplemental milk are left in tube-feeding devices or bottles.

# Feeding Plans

Three of the most common unwanted outcomes in breastfed late preterm infants are hyperbilirubinemia (jaundice), hypoglycemia (low blood sugar), and weight loss. Four preventive goals can help reduce jaundice-related complications (Hubbard et al., 2007).

1. **Optimize breastmilk intake by feeding the infant at least eight times per 24 hours and optimally 10 to 12 feedings each day, assuring that the baby is swallowing colostrum/ milk at these feedings.** This is especially important before on the onset of copious milk production. The more breast-feedings newborns experience, the lower the bilirubin levels and percentage of weight loss, and the higher the defecation frequency (Hassan & Zakerihamidi, 2018).

   Frequent feeds do not assure adequate intake unless the baby is actually swallowing during most of the feeding. Check that the baby has a deep latch, add alternate massage/breast compressions, and use a nipple shield if weak sucking pressure prevents good intake and other interventions do not seem to be effective. Some late preterm infants, especially those born at 34-35 weeks may need extra calorie supplementation. A simple breastfeeding plan can be used by the mother (Table 11).

   If the infant is unable to transfer colostrum/milk, then colostrum and or milk should be expressed and fed to the infant frequently (Figure 20).

2. **Promote quick meconium clearance.** In addition to more frequent feedings and the intake of more colostrum/milk, infant massage is an effective intervention for neonatal jaundice (Lei et al., 2018). A simple abdominal massage, such as the "I love you" pattern, is easy to teach and pleasurable to the infant (Figure 21).

**Table 11.** Sample Breastfeeding Plan for Mothers

| The Plan | Details |
|---|---|
| Feed your baby frequently | • Within 1 hour after birth<br><br>• Once every hour for the next 3 to 4 hours<br><br>• Every 2 to 3 hours until 12 hours of age<br><br>• At least 8 times each 24 hours during the hospital stay |
| Place baby skin-to-skin on your chest | |
| Watch for rapid eye movements under the eyelids (baby will wake easily) | |
| Move baby to breast when baby shows feeding cues | • Sucking movements of the mouth and tongue<br><br>• Rapid eye movements under the eyelids<br><br>• Hand-to-mouth movements<br><br>• Body movements<br><br>• Small sounds |
| Make sure you know how to tell when baby is swallowing | • Baby's jaw drops and holds for a second<br><br>• You hear a "ca" sound<br><br>• You feel a drawing action on the areola and see it move towards baby's mouth<br><br>• You hear baby swallow<br><br>• You feel the swallow when you place a finger on baby's throat<br><br>• Your nurse hears the swallow when a stethoscope is placed on baby's throat |
| Use alternate massage if baby doesn't swallow after every 1 to 3 sucks | Massage and squeeze the breast each time baby stops between sucks. This helps get more colostrum into her and keeps her sucking longer |

**Figure 20.**  Hand expressing colostrum into a spoon.
From *The Breastfeeding Atlas,* 4th ed., Wilson-Clay & Hoover, 2008.

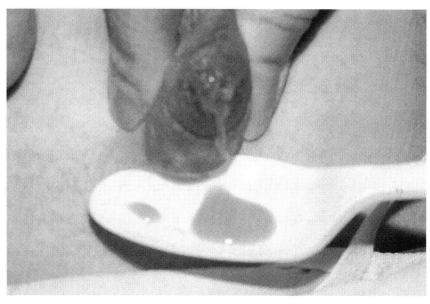

**Figure 21.** "I love you" abdominal massage.
https://www.johnsonsbaby.co.uk/baby-massage/six-weeks-plus-massage-guide

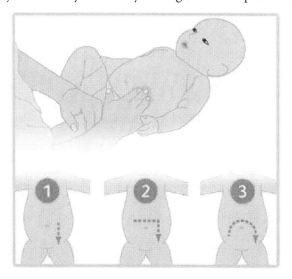

Meconium is a large reservoir for bilirubin and the quicker it can be eliminated the more likely that bilirubin will not reach excessive levels.

3. **Increase stool volume elimination.** This can happen with frequent colostrum feeds and infant abdominal massage. Larger stool volume elimination reduces the reuptake of bilirubin that can eventually wind up back in circulation.

4. **Preventing excessive weight loss is important because as the weight goes down, bilirubin levels go up.** Ensure that feedings are not missed or skipped due to ineffective feeding, the presence of visitors, or excessive interruptions. Nurses or lactation consultants should observe one feeding per shift to document that swallowing is taking place and that the mother can state when her baby is swallowing milk. Some infants may demonstrate a relatively sizeable weight loss as they diurese excessive fluid accumulated when the mother has received large amounts of IV fluid during labor or when they expel large meconium stools. This does not mean that the infant has lost an excessive amount of weight or that supplementation should be started if feeding parameters are optimal. Some hospitals use the 24-hour weight as the reference for calculation of weight loss to account for an inflated birth weight due to transplacental passage of maternal intrapartum intravenous fluids (Deng & McLaren, 2018).

## Hypoglycemia

The threat of hypoglycemia looms over the population of late preterm infants. It is beneficial to include the following in a care and feeding plan.

• Keep the infant in skin-to-skin contact with the mother for at least the first hour following birth, and consider implementing skin to skin beyond the first hour for as long as possible during the blood glucose monitoring period. A protocol that kept late preterm infants in uninterrupted skin-to-skin contact for the first two hours following birth, and up to 12 hours thereafter, reported a significant decrease in NICU admissions and IV dextrose boluses, and an increase in exclusive breastfeeding at discharge (Chiruvolu et al., 2017). Skin-to-skin care also decreases crying and stress in newborns, which further contribute to hypoglycemia.

- Avoid chilling the infant, especially by delaying the first bath until at least 12 hours post birth.

- Provide a source of carbohydrate (colostrum) on a more continuous basis during the first 12 hours rather than just bolus breastfeeds. Tozier (2013) conducted a study that included collecting colostrum not only prenatally but periodically expressed during labor and storing the drops of colostrum in feeding syringes placed on ice or in the patient's refrigerator. The infants were breastfed and provided with expressed colostrum between breastfeedings. Post-birth colostrum collection continued along with frequent feeds at breast. Colostrum collected and fed in this manner stabilized glucose levels as effectively as formula during first six hours after birth in this study. This more constant pattern of colostrum provision attempts to closely mimic the continuous supply of glucose that infants receive in utero.

- Rather than using infant formula to raise blood glucose levels, the administration of 40% glucose gel applied to the infant's buccal mucosa decreases NICU admissions due to hypoglycemia, improves breastfeeding rates, and avoids breastfeeding failure associated with maternal/infant separation (Harris et al., 2013). The use of a glucose gel intervention is cost effective for the hospital and did not prolong the infant's length of stay (Makker et al., 2018). A recent study found that the glucose concentration increases significantly after a gel application (mean increase by 11.7 mg/dL [95% CI: 10.4–12.8]) and that breastfeeding is associated with a reduced requirement of repeat gel treatment (Harris et al., 2017).

- Some late preterm infants (especially those of higher gestational ages) may do well with cue-based feedings, signaling to feed frequently and well enough to ingest adequate amounts of milk. However, not all late preterm infants will thrive using the highly flexible feeding patterns seen in full-term breastfeeding infants. They may need more of a semi-structured feeding plan, as some may not be able to make up the necessary volumes of milk when left to sleep for long periods of time. An infant left to sleep for 5 hours a couple of times each day may quickly fall behind and not be able to make up the needed volume of milk after so many hours of sleep.

- Use of behavioral feeding cues that indicate when an infant is behaviorally available to feed may be a more prudent approach. Mothers can be taught five feeding cues to indicate feeding readiness in a sleepy baby: rapid eye movements under the eyelids, hand-to-mouth movements, sucking movements of the mouth and tongue, whole body movements, and small sounds. If the baby is also being held skin to skin, these feeding cues are easier for the mother to recognize. Breastfeeding attempts when the infant indicates a lighter sleep state or alert state (which may be few) increases the chance of a more successful feeding.

Clinicians and parents may find it beneficial to create an individualized breastfeeding plan for use following discharge. A sample plan appears in Table 12. It can and should be modified to best provide parents with the tools they need to successfully breastfeed their babies.

**Table 12.** Sample Plan for Breastfeeding Your Late Preterm Infant

Breastfeeding and your milk are very important to your late preterm baby. Even though your baby may look full-term, he/she is not fully developed and may need some extra help learning to breastfeed. Your milk contains ingredients that provide protection from disease and help promote your baby's brain development that was interrupted by an early birth. Your baby may tire easily before a feeding is finished and may seem to sleep a lot. These guidelines will help get breastfeeding off to a good start.

Feed your baby on cue 8-12 times each 24 hours. Early babies are not always reliable in telling you when they need to feed. Sleeping is not an indication that baby is getting enough. Use the following cues to tell you when to start a feeding, as this is when he is ready and available:

• Rapid eye movements under the eyelids

• Sucking movements of the mouth and tongue

• Hand-to-mouth movements

• Body movements

• Small sounds (crying is a late sign of hunger and baby may not feed well)

Place your baby in a clutch or cross cradle position.

As your baby latches on, make sure his mouth is wide open.

You should hear or feel your baby swallowing every 1-3 sucks during most of the feeding.

Use alternate massage on each breast at each feeding to keep baby sucking and increase the amount of milk he receives at each feeding. Thoroughly massage and compress each part of the breast so that milk does not back up and set the stage for an infection.

If you are not sure how much milk he is getting at each feeding, you can weigh baby before and after a feeding. This will help you know if you need to offer a supplement.

Record each feeding, whether a supplement is used, the amount of pumped milk, the number of wet diapers, and the number of bowel movements on your feeding log until baby is reliably feeding and gaining weight.

If your baby does not latch to the breast, try the following:

- Gently roll your nipple between your fingers to make it easier for the baby to grasp.

- As you bring your baby to breast, have a helper place a tube feeding device or dropper in the corner of the baby's mouth and deliver a small amount of milk as the baby attempts to latch. If the baby swallows and attempts to latch again, another small amount of milk can be given. Repeat until baby no longer attempts to latch. These practice sessions should not last longer than 10 minutes to avoid tiring both you and your baby.

- Finish the feeding by finger or cup feeding.

- If the attempts at latching do not work, you may find that a silicone nipple shield will allow the baby to latch and sustain sucking at the breast. Moisten the shield with warm water, turn almost inside-out as you apply it to the breast, apply a little breastmilk to the outside of the shield, hand express milk into the shield tunnel, and bring the baby to breast. If the baby latches, continue using alternate massage throughout the feeding.

Baby should have at least 6 wet diapers and 3 or more bowel movements each day by the 5th day. Bowel movements should start turning yellow by day 4. Meconium diapers on day 5 may indicate that baby is not getting enough milk. Uric acid crystals (red stains) on day 4 in wet diapers may also indicate that baby is not transferring enough milk at the breast.

Take your baby to his physician's office 2 days after coming home from the hospital for a weight check and to make sure he is not jaundiced. A weight check every 3 days or so assures that your baby continues to gain about 1/2 to 1 ounce per day.

If baby cannot feed long enough at each feeding or is not gaining well, supplements of expressed breastmilk can be given by tube feeding at the breast, finger feeding, cup feeding, or bottle feeding. If you do not have enough milk to use as a supplement, a hydrolyzed formula can be used until your milk production has increased.

Continue to pump your milk 2 to 3 times each day to use as a supplement and to improve your milk supply. Try "power pumping" once or twice each day. Pump for 5 to 10 minutes until the milk stops spraying from the first let down. Wait 15 to 20 minutes and pump again until the milk stops spraying. Almost half of the milk that is available in the breast is pumped with the first let down. Power pumping takes advantage of these "first" letdowns to mimic frequent feedings and helps increase your milk production. Depending on how your baby is doing at the breast, pumping should continue until he is 40-42 weeks corrected age, weaning off the pump over the first month home.

# Initiating and Maintaining Maternal Milk Supply

The first 7 to 14 days following delivery are important for establishing an abundant milk supply. Milk production at 4 to 7 days is related to milk production and adequacy at 6 weeks after birth, for mothers of both healthy breastfeeding term infants and non-nursing preterm infants (Hill & Aldag, 2005). Feedings at the breast or expressing should begin within the first hour after delivery (Parker et al., 2015).

One method to maximize milk production when the infant is either ineffective at feeding directly from the breast or is separated or unable to directly nurse is to begin by using the following protocol (Morton et al., 2009).

- Begin double pumping (pumping both breasts simultaneously) within the first 6 hours (preferably during the first hour).

- Pump eight times per day for 15 minutes.

- Add hand expression of colostrum as frequently as possible during the first three days.

- After the onset of copious milk production, pump eight or more times per day until only drops can be expressed

- While pumping, mothers simultaneously massage and compress the breast.

- When milk flow stops, pumping stops, and the breasts are massaged again.

- Following this massage, hand expression or pumping is performed using whichever method is more effective at removing residual milk.

The above bullet points are referred to as hands-on pumping. Mothers who used hand expression more than five times per day during the first three days following birth had milk volumes that exceeded the average intake (812 mL/day) of 3-month-old breastfed term babies. Milk production should be carefully watched during the first 14 days. The goal is to produce 3500 mL/week-118 ounces (500 mL/day-16 ounces) by the end of the second week to achieve optimal output for sustained lactation (Hill et al., 1999).

This is important if the mother is exclusively pumping. Milk volumes that reach 800-1000 mL/24 hours by 10 to 14 days provide a reserve such that if the maternal milk supply drops by as much as 50% during the infant's hospitalization, sufficient volume will remain to adequately nourish the baby once discharged from the hospital (Hurst & Meier, 2005). Pumping will continue until the infant is able to consume adequate volumes of milk directly from the breast, or to use as a supplement should the infant continue to experience difficulty with direct breastfeeding.

Maternal stress at having a late preterm infant is often increased by concerns about having an adequate milk supply. When considering a breast pump to initiate or increase milk supply, it is important that mothers secure a high quality, multi-user breast pump capable of expressing milk simultaneously from both breasts. The flange or breast shield should be properly fitted, as nipples swell during pumping (Wilson-Clay & Hoover, 2002). If the nipple becomes strangulated in the flange tunnel, soreness, reduced milk flow, and low milk supply can result. Standard pump kits usually provide flanges whose nipple tunnel opening is 24 mm to 25 mm, but some mothers may benefit from flanges with a larger opening.

There is no standard protocol for milk insufficiency. Before recommending any galactagogue, it is important to ascertain, as best as possible, what is contributing to low milk production and start with the primary means of increasing overall milk production (frequent and adequate removal of milk from the breasts). In addition, evaluate other medical factors that may potentially be involved (Brodribb & the Academy of Breastfeeding Medicine, 2018).

Faltering milk production can herald the abandonment of breast-feeding. This frustrating situation may be helped by several interventions:

- **Additional pumping sessions may be advised but this may be limited, depending on individual situations.** If more pumping sessions cannot be added, then more effective pumping suggestions may be warranted. Power pumping is a short-term strategy suggested by lactation consultant Catherine Watson Genna (Marasco & West, 2020). It has various versions that involve pumping for a short period of time (5 to 10 minutes), stopping, and restarting pumping 15 or 20 minutes later, doing this several times in an hour, several times a day, for several days until the milk output increases. This takes advantage of the first let down of milk, which can release almost half of the volume of milk in the breast (Ramsay et al., 2006), with multiple "first" let-downs in an hour.

- **Preparations such as domperidone and metoclopramide are the more commonly discussed pharmaceutical galactagogues.** Domperidone has been shown to have good evidence for a moderate short-term increase in milk supply, but should be avoided in women with an increased risk for QTc-prolongation (cardiac arrhythmia) (Grzeskowiak et al., 2019). Mothers with a history of cardiac arrhythmia or taking medications that inhibit the metabolism of domperidone (fluconazole, erythromycin) should avoid domperidone.

- Domperidone is not available in the United States except occasionally from a compounding pharmacy with a prescription.

There is weak evidence that domperidone might be slightly more effective than metoclopramide, but metoclopramide crosses the blood-brain barrier and has a risk for depression, tardive dyskinesia, and other central nervous system side effects. Metoclopramide should not be used longer than five days.

- **Lactogenic foods and herbal galactagogues have been recommended and used for centuries. Some have scant evidence for their efficacy and others with more data to support their use.** Herbal galactagogues work in different ways, depending on what is contributing to low milk production. This is why some may be of no benefit and others might be helpful. With the use of herbal or culinary remedies, it is important to determine the cause of the low milk production first, if possible, and target the herbs with properties that might more closely address the issue. A good resource is the book book is "*Making More Milk*, 2nd edition" by Marasco and West (2020).

- **Acupuncture has been used in Traditional Chinese Medicine (TCM) to treat low milk production for a couple of thousand years.** It can increase both prolactin and oxytocin and has also been used to treat low thyroid levels and fertility issues. While studies may use different acupuncture points, this intervention has been shown to be quite effective in increasing milk production (He et al., 2008; Jiang, 2014; Wang et al., 2007; Xian, 2017). It may be a worthwhile approach for some parents to investigate.

- **Acupressure is a technique that uses fingertip or thumb pressure applied to specific acupoints in the body, depending on the desired outcome.** It has been taught to mothers to perform on themselves and successfully increased milk volume in mothers with decreased milk production (Esfahani et al., 2015).

- **Acupoint-tuina therapy is an ancient form of medical massage in Chinese medicine.** In a study that included finger massage of various body areas, as well as on both breasts for the first two days postpartum, milk volume was significantly increased, as well as prolactin levels (Lu et al., 2019).

- **Auricular therapy uses specific sticking points on the ear to affect health outcomes.** It has been shown to be another form of Chinese medicine that can increase milk production (Zhou et al., 2009).

- **Another low-tech intervention for milk insufficiency is reflexology, which focuses on trigger points in the foot.** Increased milk production was seen in preterm mothers and those who had undergone a cesarean delivery after reflexology points were stimulated on the foot (Mirzaie et al., 2018; Mohammadpour et al., 2018).

- **The warming of tissues is a known therapeutic intervention that increases local blood flow and metabolism in tissues. It facilitates excretion of tissue waste materials and phago-cytosis, and enhances tissue nutrition.** Warm compresses placed on the breasts has long been recommended to aid the let-down reflex. Yigit et al. (2012) studied if warming the breast prior to pumping would increase the volume of milk expressed from a warmed breast compared with the other breast, which was not warmed. Mothers placed a warm com-press (40.5C/104.9F) on one breast prior to pumping with an electric breast pump. The amount of milk obtained from the warmed breasts was significantly higher than that obtained from the non-warmed breasts. This is a simple intervention that may increase milk yields.

- **Kent et al. (2011) found that warmed pump flanges resulted in decreased time to remove 80% of the total milk yield and increased the percentage of available milk removed after 5 minutes of expression.** This increase in pumping efficiency may be welcomed by time-stressed families.

- **Keith et al. (2012) found that preterm pump-dependent mothers who listened to special flute music during the first week of lactation for 30 minutes while pumping produced significantly more milk, with a higher fat content, compared with mothers who did not listen to the music.** Soothing music increases oxytocin levels (Nilsson, 2009), improves endothelial vasoreactivity, and lowers stress and cortisol levels.

- **Therapeutic taping, often seen on athletes and used in sports medicine, is designed to assist in fluid movement by increasing blood flow and drainage of tissues.** In a small study of mothers with low milk supply, Kinesiotape® was applied to the breasts using fan cuts for relaxing the pectoralis muscles and facilitating fluid movement. Mothers reported doubling or tripling the amount of milk they could pump after the tape was applied (Valdez et al., 2018).

# Conclusion

Assisting the family of a late preterm infant in their breastfeeding journey can be time consuming and frustrating. It will call upon the clinician's assessment skills and knowledge base of breastfeeding in special situations. The health benefits of breastfeeding and/or the provision of mother's own milk until the infant is established at the breast validate the increased use of health provider time to see that this happens. Because it is an investment in health that lasts a lifetime, it is worth the time, effort, and patience.

# Test Questions

## Breastfeeding the Late Preterm Infant
Marsha Walker, RN, IBCLC

1. Babies who are born "just a little early" or "near term" often have their unique vulnerabilities overlooked.

   a. True

   b. False

2. When reporting the gestational age of a late preterm infant:

   a. It should be rounded off to the nearest completed week

   b. It will help parents and clinicians anticipate what to expect

   c. It typically includes both the number of weeks plus days

   d. All of the above

3. Babies born at 37 to 38 weeks are no more likely than term babies to be admitted to the NICU.

   a. True

   b. False

4.  **According to the nomenclature of prematurity, the gestational age of a late preterm infant is:**

    a. 32 to 33 weeks

    b. 34 to 36 weeks

    c. 37 to 38 weeks

    d. 40 to 41 weeks

5.  **A baby born at 37 weeks would be called:**

    a. Preterm

    b. Late preterm

    c. Early term

    d. None of the above

6.  **Which of the following maternal conditions contribute to the risk of late preterm and early term deliveries?**

    a. Diabetes

    b. Hypertension

    c. Inflammation

    d. Infection

    e. All of the above

7.  **Which of the following is not associated with late preterm delivery?**

    a. Resuscitation at delivery

    b. Shorter length of birth hospitalization

    c. Feeding difficulties

    d. Mortality

8.  **According to Kuzniewicz et al. (2013), some of the most common reasons for hospital readmission include all of the following except:**

    a. Sepsis

    b. Jaundice

    c. Feeding problems

    d. Allergies

9.  **What is the best description of the brain of a late preterm or early term baby?**

    a. Just a smaller version of a term baby's brain

    b. Has the same maturation level as a term infant

    c. Can easily coordinate suck/swallow/feed

    d. Has experienced an interruption in development

10. **Breastmilk is especially important for the developing brain of the late preterm and early term infants. Which of the following components of breastmilk support brain development?**

    a. Sialic acid

    b. Lactose

    c. Human milk oligosaccharide 2`

    d. All of the above

11. **Fetal Hypoxia is the lack of:**

    a. Protein

    b. Oxygen

    c. Hydration

    d. all of the above

12. **Limitations on milk volume may predispose the late preterm infant to an even higher risk of:**

    a. dehydration

    b. hypoglycemia

    c. jaundice

    d. all of the above

13. Women with a low pre-pregnancy body mass index have a higher rate of delayed lactogenesis than women with a high BMI.

   a. True

   b. False

14. Skin-to-skin is an important strategy in the prevention of which of the following?

   a. Hypothermia

   b. Frequent urination

   c. Childhood obesity

   d. Tuberculosis

15. If the infant has diminished muscle tone, providing extra jaw support from the _____ hand position may help stabilize the jaw such that the infant does not keep slipping off of the nipple or does not bite or clench the jaw to keep from sliding off the breast.

   a. Clutch

   b. Dancer

   c. Prancer

   d. All of the above

16. **The newborn period is a critical developmental window of time where the brain and nervous system are especially sensitive to certain environmental stimuli.**

    a. True

    b. False

17. **Which of these does NOT cause the baby to "shut down?"**

    a. Bright lights

    b. Loud noises

    c. Skin-to-skin contact

    d. Talking

18. **The first _____ following delivery are very important for establishing an abundant milk supply.**

    a. 3 hours

    b. 2 days

    c. 7 to 14 days

    d. 12 months

Send your test answers to
**info@praeclaruspress.com** in order
to receive your certificate.
Questions and concerns: **ken@praecaruspress.com**

# Resources for Parents

## Booklet

*Breastfeeding your late preterm baby*

Best Start Resource Centre: Ontario's Maternal Newborn and Early Child Development Resource Centre

Also available in: French, Arabic, Bengali, Chinese, Farsi, Gujarati, Hindi, Korean, Punjabi, Russian, Serbian, Somali, Spanish, Tagalog, Tamil, Urdu, and Vietnamese.

https://resources.beststart.org/product/b26e-breastfeeding-your-late-preterm-baby-booklet/

## Books

Casemore, S. (2014). *Exclusively pumping breastmilk: A guide to providing expressed breast milk for your baby, 2nd Ed.* Napanee, Ontario, Canada: Gray Lion Publishing.

Marasco L., & West, D. (2020). *Making more milk, 2nd Ed.* New York, McGraw-Hill.

## Apps

*My NICU baby app*
https://www.marchofdimes.org/nicufamilysupport/my-nicu-baby-app.aspx

*Pacify*
www. https://www.pacify.com/

# Video

*Getting started with breastfeeding*

Stanford Medicine, Newborn Nursery

https://med.stanford.edu/newborns/professional-education/
breastfeeding.html

# Where to find help

*Find an IBCLC Lactation Consultant and Other Breastfeeding Support*

United States Lactation Consultant Association

https://uslca.org/resources/find-an-ibclc

*ZipMilk*

Massachusetts Breastfeeding Coalition

www.zipmilk.org

# Glossary

**Alternate massage/breast compressions** - Mother massages and compresses breast each time baby pauses between sucking bursts. This reduces the effort needed by the baby to withdraw milk from the breast. All quadrants of each breast need to be massaged and compressed during each feeding to prevent milk stasis and lowered milk production from inadequate drainage.

**Apnea** - Brief pauses in breathing.

**Areolar compression/reverse pressure softening** - Mother presses fingers around areola to make indentations or pits that serve to expose the nipple, making it easier for baby to latch to an engorged areola.

**Biological nurturing** - Mother holds late preterm infants so that the baby's chest, abdomen, and legs are closely flexed around her body and unrestricted access to the breast is offered. It has been proposed that the preterm infant can continue to be incubated or gestated in the mother's arms during the early days following a late preterm birth.

**Bradycardia** - A slow heartbeat which results in the heart not being able to pump enough blood to provide oxygen to the body.

**Brown fat** - Fat in newborn mammals used to generate body heat.

**Buccinator muscles** - Thin, flat muscle forming the wall of the cheek.

**Cephalhematoma** - A blood cyst, tumor, or swelling of the scalp of a newborn due to seeping of blood beneath the skin, often resulting from birth trauma.

**Cup feeding** - Infant is fed using a medicine cup. The medicine cup with a small amount of milk is placed against the infant's lower lip. The cup is tipped so that the milk is available to the infant when his tongue protrudes. The infant slowly sips or laps the milk.

**Dancer hand position** - Mother supports baby's chin during breastfeeding so that baby does not slip off nipple or bite or clench jaws to keep from sliding off breast.

**Digital infant scale** - Scale used to weigh infant before and after feeding to determine amount ingested during the feed.

**Early term infant** - Infant born between 37 0/7 weeks and 38 6/7 weeks.

**Finger feeding** - Infant is fed using a tube taped or held to a feeder's finger. The feeder's finger is placed pad side up and the infant is encouraged to draw the finger into his mouth. A small amount of milk is delivered through the tube when the infant sucks.

**Half-life** - Time required for half of a dose of a drug to be metabolized or eliminated from the body.

**Hypoglycemia** - Low blood sugar.

**Hypothermia** - Low body temperature.

**Hypotonia** - Low muscle tone.

**Iatrogenic preterm birth** - Elective delivery of preterm infants.

**Jaundice** - Condition that results when bilirubin levels increase in the blood, resulting in yellowish staining of the eyes and skin. Extremely high levels in an infant can cause neurologic damage and possibly death.

**Kernicterus** - Chronic and permanent clinical outcomes of bilirubin toxicity, including athetoid cerebral palsy, hearing loss, paralysis of upward gaze, dental dysplasia, and possibly intellectual handicaps.

**Lactose** - A disaccharide found in milk composed of glucose and galactose-milk sugar.

**Late preterm infant** - Infant born between 34 0/7 weeks and 36 6/7 weeks.

**Mandible** - Lower jaw

**Masseter muscle** - Muscle involved in chewing, biting, swallowing, and speech.

**Morbidity** – Illness

**Mortality** – Death

**Muscles involved in moving tongue:**

    **Styloglossus muscles** - Small, short muscles located on each side of the tongue that links the sides of the tongue to the base of the skull. Contraction of these two muscles pulls the tongue back and up.

    **Palatoglossus muscles** - Muscles that originate from the soft palate and insert on each side of the tongue. These muscles work together to raise the back of the tongue.

    **Genioglossus muscles** - Flat, triangular muscles that originate from the inner surface of the front of the lower jaw and the hyoid bone and insert on each side of the tip of the tongue. When the two muscles contract at the same time, the tongue is protruded by its whole foundation being pulled forward.

    **Hyoglossus muscles** - Thin, flat strap of muscle located on each side of the tongue. It originates from the side of the hyoid bone in the throat and passes vertically inside the tongue. When the two hyoglossus muscles contract, they depress the tongue and turn the sides down.

    The genioglossus, styloglossus, palatoglossus, and hyoglossus muscles work together to move the tongue.

**Myelination** - Coating of the branches of nerve cells with a fatty substance to keep ions from leaking out. This coating speeds transmission of electrical signals along a nerve fiber.

**Necrotizing enterocolitis (NEC)** - Medical condition primarily seen in premature infants. NEC involves infection and inflammation that causes destruction of the bowel or part of the bowel.

**Nipple tug** - Gentle tug on the nipple (or can pull baby slightly away) while infant is latched on, causing baby to draw the nipple/areola farther back into his mouth to maintain latch.

**Nomogram** - Graph that looks at the infant's gestational age, age in hours post birth, and bilirubin level to predict the likelihood of severe jaundice.

**Oligosaccharides** - Carbohydrate molecule composed of 3-20 simple sugars (monosaccharides).

**Oropharynx** - The part of the throat at the back of the mouth. It includes the soft palate, the base of the tongue, and the tonsils.

**Paced feeding** - Bottle feeding where feeder regulates infant suck/swallow/pauses by removing the nipple from the infant's mouth after every 3 to 5 sucks, allowing a 3-5 second pause for breathing. The nipple rests on the midpoint of the infant's upper lip during the pause, allowing the infant to draw the nipple back into the mouth when ready to resume feeding. With late preterm infants, the bottle can be tipped downward to stop the flow of liquid into the baby's mouth, giving the infant time to swallow and breathe.

**Periventricular Leukomalacia (PVL)** - Death of white matter of the brain due to softening of the brain tissue. This is caused by a lack of oxygen or blood flow to the periventricular area of the brain, by bleeding into the brain, or by a bacterial infection in mother or infant that triggers a cytokine response in the brain.

**Post term infant** - Infant born at 42 weeks or beyond.

**Power pumping** - Method of pumping to increase milk supply. Mothers pump for 5-10 minutes or until milk stops spraying from first let down, then wait 15-20 minutes and pump again until milk stops spraying. Power pumping takes advantage of first letdowns to mimic frequent feeding and helps increase milk production.

**PREEMIE ACT** - Legislation passed in 2006 that mandates research expansion, better provider education and training, and a Surgeon General's conference to address the growing epidemic of preterm births.

**Retinopathy of prematurity** - Potentially blinding eye disorder that primarily affects premature infants weighing less than 2 3/4 pounds or born before 31 weeks of gestation.

**Sepsis** - Over reaction by the body to an infection.

**Sialic acid** – A chemical component of a number of complex chemical structures in the human body. A disturbance in sialic acid metabolism may lead to a concentration of sialic acid in the blood, urine or solid tissue. This almost always leads to physical and mental deterioration.

**Subcutaneous fat** - Fatty or adipose tissue that lies directly under the skin.

**Sublingual pressure** - Mother slips index finger directly behind and under the tip of the chin where the tongue attaches, limiting downward movement of the jaw so that suction is not broken each time the jaw drops.

**Temporalis muscle** - Muscle responsible for raising the mandible.

**Term infant** - Infant born between 39 0/7 and 41 6/7 weeks of gestation.

**Visuomotor integrative skills** - Vision and movement working together to produce actions. Some of the complications of premature birth affect development of visuomotor skills.

# References

## A

Abouelfettoh, A.M., Dowling, D.A., Dabash, S.A., Elguindy, S.R., & Seoud, I.A. (2008). Cup versus bottle feeding for hospitalized late preterm infants in Egypt: A quasi-experimental study. *International Breastfeeding Journal, 3*, 27-38.

al-Sayed, L.E., Schrank, W.I., & Thach, B.T. (1994). Ventilatory sparing strategies and swallowing pattern during bottle feeding in human infants. *Journal of Applied Physiology, 77*, 78-83.

Alatalo, D., Jiang, L., Geddes, D., & Hassanipour, F. (2020). Nipple deformation and peripheral pressure on the areola during breastfeeding. *Journal of Biomechanical Engineering, 142*, 011004. https://doi.org/10.1115/1.4043665.

Ali, U.A., & Norwitz, E.R. (2009). Vacuum-assisted vaginal delivery. *Reviews in Obstetrics and Gynecology, 2*, 5-17.

American Academy of Pediatrics, Subcommittee on Hyperbilirubinemia. (2004). Management of hyperbilirubinemia in the newborn infant 35 or more weeks of gestation. *Pediatrics, 114*, 297-316.

American College of Obstetricians and Gynecologists. (2019a). Avoidance of nonmedically indicated early-term deliveries and associated neonatal morbidities. ACOG Committee Opinion No. 765. *Obstetrics and Gynecology, 133*, e156–e163.

American College of Obstetricians and Gynecologists, (2019b). Medically indicated late-preterm and early-term deliveries. ACOG Committee Opinion No. 764. *Obstetrics and Gynecology, 133*, e151-e155.

Arthur, P.G., Smith, M., & Hartmann, P.E. (1989). Milk lactose, citrate, and glucose as markers of lactogenesis in normal and diabetic women. *Journal of Pediatric Gastroenterology and Nutrition, 9*, 488-496.

Aycicek, A., Erel, O., Kocyigit, A., Selek, S., & Demirkol, M.R. (2006). Breast milk provides better antioxidant power than does formula. *Nutrition, 22*, 616-619.

Aytekin, A., Albayrak, E.B., Kucukoglu, S., & Caner, I. (2014). The effect of feeding with spoon and bottle on the time of switching to full breastfeeding and sucking success in preterm babies. *Turkish Archives of Pediatrics, 49*, 307-313.

Azad, M.B., Moyce, B.L., Guillemette, L., Pascoe, C.D., Wicklow, B., McGavock, J.M., Halayko, A.J., & Dolinsky, V.W. (2017). Diabetes in pregnancy and lung health in offspring: Developmental origins of respiratory disease. *Paediatric Respiratory Reviews, 21*, 19-26.

# B

Babendure, J.B., Reifsnider, E., Mendias, E., Moramarco, M.W., & Davila, Y.R. (2015). Reduced breastfeeding rates among obese mothers: A review of contributing factors, clinical considerations and future directions. *International Breastfeeding Journal, 10*, 1-11.

Batista, C.L.C., Rodrigues, V.P., Ribeiro, V.S., & Nascimento, M.D.S.B. (2019). Nutritive and non-nutritive sucking patterns associated with pacifier use and bottle-feeding in full-term infants. *Early Human Development, 132*, 18-23.

Becker, G.E., Smith, H.A., & Cooney, F. (2016). Methods of milk expression for lactating women. *Cochrane Database Systematic Review*, 2016(9): CD006170.

Beilin, Y., Bodian, C.A., Weiser, J., Hossain, S., Arnold, I., Feierman, D.E., Martin, G., & Holzman, I. (2005). Effect of labor epidural analgesia with and without fentanyl on infant breast-feeding: A prospective, randomized, double-blind study. *Anesthesiology, 103, 1211-1217.*

*Belfort, M.B., Drouin, K., Riley, J.F., Gregory, K.E., Philipp, B.L., Parker, M.G., & Sen, S. (2018). Prevalence and trends in donor human milk use in the well-baby nursery: A survey of Northeast United States birth hospitals. Breastfeeding Medicine, 13, 34-41.*

Bell, A.F., White-Traut, R., & Rankin, K. (2013). Fetal exposure to synthetic oxytocin and the relationship with prefeeding cues within one hour postbirth. *Early Human Development, 89,* 137-143.

Bennett, C.F., Galloway, C., & Grassley, J.S. (2018). Education for WIC peer counselors about breastfeeding the late preterm infant. *Journal of Nutrition Education and Behavior, 50,* 198-203.

Berger, P.K., Plows, J.F., Jones, R.B., Alderete, T.L., Yonemitsu, C., Poulsen, M., Ryoo, J.H., Peterson, B.S., Bode, L., & Goran, M.I. (2020). Human milk oligosaccharide 2'-fucosyllactose links feedings at 1 month to cognitive development at 24 months in infants of normal and overweight mothers. *PLoS One, 15*(2), e0228323.

Bergman, N.J. (2013). Neonatal stomach volume and physiology suggest feeding at 1-h intervals. *Acta Paediatrica, 102,* 773-777.

Bergman, N.J. (2014). The neuroscience of birth – and the case for Zero Separation. *Curationis, 37*(2), Art. #1440.

Bhutani, V.K. (2012). Late preterm infants: Major cause of prematurity and adverse outcomes of neonatal hyperbilirubinemia. *Indian Pediatrics, 49,* 704-705.

Boies, E.G., & Vaucher, Y.E. (2016). ABM clinical protocol #10: Breastfeeding the late preterm (34-36 6/7 weeks of gestation) and early term infants (37-38 6/7 weeks of gestation), second revision 2016. *Breastfeeding Medicine, 11,* 494-500.

Briere, C-E., Lucas, R., McGrath, J.M., Lussier, M., & Brownell, E. (2015). Establishing breastfeeding with the late preterm infant in the NICU. *Journal of Obstetric, Gynecologic, and Neonatal Nursing, 44,* 102-113.

Brimdyr, K., Cadwell, K., Widstrom, A-M., Svensson, K., Neumann, M., Hart, E.A., Harrington, S., & Phillips, R. (2015). The association between common labor drugs and suckling when skin-to-skin during the first hour after birth. *Birth, 42*, 319-328.

Brimdyr, K., Cadwell, K., Widstrom, A-M., Svensson, K., & Phillips, R. (2019). The effect of labor medications on normal newborn behavior in the first hour after birth: A prospective cohort study. *Early Human Development, 132*, 30-36.

Brodribb, W., & the Academy of Breastfeeding Medicine. (2018). ABM clinical protocol #9: use of galactogogues in initiating or augmenting maternal milk production, second revision 2018. *Breastfeeding Medicine, 13*, 307-314.

Brown, A., & Jordan, S. (2013). Impact of birth complications on breastfeeding duration: An internet survey. *Journal of Advanced Nursing, 69*, 828–839.

Brown, H.K., Speechley, K.N., Macnab, J., Natale, R., & Campbell, M.K. (2015). Biological determinants of spontaneous later preterm and early term birth: A retrospective cohort study. *British Journal of Obstetrics and Gynecology, 122*, 491-499.

# C

Cannon, A.M., Sakalidis, V.S., Lai, C.T., Perrella, S.L., & Geddes, D.T. (2016). Vacuum characteristics of the sucking cycle and relationships with milk removal from the breast in term infants. *Early Human Development, 96*, 1-6.

Chan, E., Leong, P., Malouf, R., & Quigley, M.A. (2016). Long-term cognitive and school outcomes of late preterm and early term infants: A systematic review. *Child: Care, Health and Development, 42*, 297-312.

Chichlowski M, De Lartigue, G., German, J.B., Raybould, H.E., & Mills, D.A. (2012). Bifidobacteria isolated from infants and cultured on human milk oligosaccharides affect intestinal epithelial function. Journal of Pediatric Gastroenterology Nutrition, 55, 321–327.

Chiruvolu, A., Miklis, K.K., Stanzo, K.C., Petrey, B., Groves, C.G., McCord, K., Qin, H., Desai, S., & Tolia, V.N. (2017). Effects of skin-to-skin care on late preterm and term infants at-risk for neonatal hypoglycemia. *Pediatric Quality and Safety, 2*, e030.

Christensson, K., Siles, C., Moreno, L., Belaustequi, A., De La Fuente, P., Lagercrantz, H., Puyol, P., & Winberg, J. (1992). Temperature, metabolic adaption and crying in healthy full-term newborns cared for skin-to-skin or in a cot. *Acta Paediatrica, 81*, 488-493.

Colson, S. (2014). Does the mother's posture have a protective role to play during skin-to-skin care? *Clinical Lactation, 5*, 41-49.

Colson S.D., Meek, J.H., & Hawdon, J.M. (2008). Optimal positions for the release of primitive neonatal reflexes stimulating breastfeeding. *Early Human Development, 84*, 441-449.

Committee on Fetus and Newborn. (2011). Postnatal glucose homeostasis in late-preterm and term infants. *Pediatrics, 127*, 575-579.

Cotterman, K.J. (2004). Reverse pressure softening: a simple tool to prepare areola for easier latching during engorgement. *Journal of Human Lactation, 20*, 227-237.

Crenshaw J. T., Cadwell K., Brimdyr K., Widström A., Svensson K., Champion J. D., & Winslow E. H. (2012). Use of a video-ethnographic intervention (PRECESS Immersion Method) to improve skin-to-skin care and breastfeeding rates. *Breastfeeding Medicine, 7*(2), 69–78.

Csaszar-Nagy, N., & Bokkon, I. (2018). Mother-newborn separation at birth in hospitals: A possible risk for neurodevelopmental disorders? *Neuroscience and Biobehavioral Reviews, 84*, 337-351.

Cullinane, M., Amir, L.H., Donath, S.M., Garland, S.M., Tabrizi, S.N., Payne, M.S., & Bennett, C.M. (2015). Determinants of mastitis in women in the CASTLE study: a cohort study. *BMC Family Practice, 16*, 181.

# D

Danner, S.C., & Cerutti, E.R. (1984). *Nursing your neurologically impaired baby.* Rochester, NY: Childbirth Graphics.

DeBortoli, J., & Amir, L.H. (2016). Is onset of lactation delayed in women with diabetes in pregnancy? A systematic review. *Diabetes Medicine, 33*, 17-24.

Delnord, M., & Zeitlin, J. (2019). Epidemiology of late preterm and early term births – An international perspective. *Seminars in Fetal and Neonatal Medicine, 24*, 3-10.

Demirci, J.R., Happ, M.B., Bogen, D.L., Albrecht, S.A., & Cohen, S.M. (2015). Weighing worth against uncertain work: The interplay of exhaustion, ambiguity, hope and disappointment in mothers breastfeeding late preterm infants. *Maternal Child Nutrition, 11*, 59-72.

Deng, X., & McLaren, M. (2018). Using 24-hour weight as reference for weight loss calculation reduces supplementation and promotes exclusive breastfeeding in infants born by cesarean section. Breastfeeding Medicine, 13, 128-134.

Deoni, S.C.L., Dean, D.C., Piryatinsky, I., O'Muircheartaigh, J., Waskiewicz, N., Lehman, K., Han, M., & Dirks, H. (2013). Breastfeeding and early white matter development: A cross-sectional study. *Neuroimage, 82*, 77-86.

Dewey, K.G. (2001). Maternal and fetal stress are associated with impaired lactogenesis in humans. *Journal of Nutrition, 131*, 3012S-3015S.

Dewey, K.G., Nommsen-Rivers, L.A., Heinig, M.J., & Cohen, R.J. (2003). Risk factors for suboptimal infant breastfeeding behavior, delayed onset of lactation, and excess neonatal weight loss. *Pediatrics, 112*(3 Pt 1), 607–619.

DiCioccio, H.C., Ady, C., Bena, J.F., & Albert, N.M. (2019). Initiative to improve exclusive breastfeeding by delaying the newborn bath. *Journal of Obstetric, Gynecologic & Neonatal Nursing, 48*, 189-196.

Dimitraki, M., Tsikouras, P., Manav, B., (2016). Evaluation of the effect of natural and emotional stress of labor on lactation and breastfeeding. *Archives of Gynecology and Obstetrics, 293,* 317-328.

Dosani, A., Hemraj, J., Premji, S.S., Currie, G., Reilly, S. M., Lodha, A.K., Young, M., & Hall. M. (2017). Breastfeeding the late preterm infant: Experiences of mothers and perceptions of public health nurses. *International Breastfeeding Journal, 12,* 23.

Dowling, D.A., Meier, P.P., Di Fiore, J.M., Blatz, M., & Martin, R.J. (2002). Cup-feeding for preterm infants: Mechanics and safety. *Journal of Human Lactation, 18,* 13-20.

# E

Edgehouse L, Radzyminski SG. (1990). A device for supplementing breast-feeding. *MCN American Journal of Maternal Child Nursing, 15,* 34-35.

Eglash, A., Ziemer, A.L., & Chevalier, A. (2010). Health professionals' attitudes and use of nipple shields for breastfeeding women. *Breastfeeding Medicine, 5,* 147-151.

El-Khuffash, A., Jain, A., Lewandowski, A.J., & Levy, P.T. (2019). Preventing disease in the 21st century: Early breast milk exposure and later cardiovascular health in premature infants. *Pediatric Research,* doi: 10.1038/s41390-019-0648-5. [ ahead of print].

Engle, W.A., Tomashek, K.M., Wallman, C., & Committee on Fetus and Newborn, American Academy of Pediatrics. (2007). "Late-preterm" infants: A population at risk. *Pediatrics, 120,* 1390-1401.

Esfahani, M.S., Berenji-Sooghe, S., Valiani, M., & Ehsanpour, S. (2015). Effect of acupressure on milk volume of breastfeeding mothers referring to selected health care centers in Tehran. *Iranian Journal of Nursing and Midwifery Research, 20,* 7-11.

# F

Ferrante, A., Silvestri, R., & Montinaro, C. (2006). The importance of choosing the right feeding aids to maintain breastfeeding after interruption. *International Journal of Orofacial Myology, 32,* 58-67.

Ferrero, D.M., Larson, J., Jacobsson, B., Di Renzo, G.C., Norman, J.E., Martin Jr., J.N…Simpson, J.L. (2016). Cross-country individual participant analysis of 4.1 million singleton births in five countries with very high human development index confirms known associations but provides no biologic explanation for 2/3 of all preterm births. *PLoS One, 11,* e0162506.

Foda, M., Kawashima, T., Nakamura, S., Kobayashi, M., & Oku, T. (2004).

Composition of milk obtained from unmassaged versus massaged breasts of lactating mothers. *Journal of Pediatric Gastroenterology and Nutrition, 38,* 484-487.

Food and Drug Administration. (2016). *Nubain.* Retrieved December 12, 2019 from https://www.accessdata.fda.gov/drugsatfda_docs/label/2016/018024s041lbl.pdf.

Forsgren, M., Isolauri, E., Salminen, S., & Rautava, S. (2017). Late preterm birth has direct and indirect effects on infant gut microbiota development during the first six months of life. *Acta Paediatrica, 106,* 1103-1109.

Fukuda, S., Toh, H., Hase, K., Oshima, K., Nakanishi, Y., Yoshimura, K., Tobe, T., Clarke, J.M., Topping, D.L., Suzuki, T., Taylor, T.D., Itoh, K., Kikuchi, J., Morita, H., Hattori, M., & Ohno, H. (2011). Bifidobacteria can protect from enteropathogenic infection through production of acetate. *Nature, 469,* 543–547.

# G

Garg, M., & Devaskar, S.U. (2006). Glucose metabolism in the late preterm infant. *Clinics in Perinatology, 33,* 853-870.

Geddes, D.T., Chooi, K., Nancarrow, K., Hepworth, A.R., Gardner, H., & Simmer, K. (2017). Characterisation of sucking dynamics of breastfeeding preterm infants: A cross sectional study. *BMC Pregnancy Childbirth 17,* 386.

Geddes, D.T., Kent, J.C., Mitoulas, L.R., & Hartmann, P.E. (2008). Tongue movement and intra-oral vacuum in breastfeeding infants. *Early Human Development, 84,* 471-477.

Gomes, C.F., Trezza, E.M.C., Murade, E.C.M., & Padovani, C.R. (2006). Surface electromyography of facial muscles during natural and artificial feeding of infants. *Journal of Pediatrics (Rio J), 82,* 103-109.

Grigoriadis, S., VonderPorten, E.H., Mamisashvili, L., Eady, A., Tomlinson, G., Dennis, C.L., Koren, G., Steiner, M., Mousmanis, P., Cheung, A., & Ross, L.E. (2013).The effect of prenatal antidepressant exposure on neonatal adaptation: a systematic review and meta-analysis. *Journal of Clinical Psychiatry, 74,* e309–e320.

Groom, K.M. (2019). Antenatal corticosteroids after 34 weeks' gestation: Do we have the evidence? *Seminars in Fetal and Neonatal Medicine, 24,* 189-196.

Grzeskowiak, L.E., Wlodek, M.E., & Geddes, D.T. (2019). What evidence do we have for pharmaceutical galactagogues in the treatment of lactation insufficiency? A narrative review. *Nutrients, 11,* E974.

Guala, A., Boscardini, L., Visentin, R., Angellotti, P., Grugni, L., Barbaglia, M., Chapin, E., Castelli, E., & Finale, E. (2017). Skin-to-skin contact in cesarean birth and duration of breastfeeding: A cohort study. *Scientific World Journal, 2017,* 1940756.

Guoth-Gumberger, M. (2006). *Breastfeeding with the supplementary nursing system (SNS)*. Retrieved from: http://www.breastfeeding-support.de/eng/pub.htm.

# H

Hall, R.T., Mercer, A.M., Teasley, S.L., McPherson, D.M., Simon, S.D., Santos, S.R., Meyers, B.M., & Hipsh, N.E. (2002). A breastfeeding assessment score to evaluate the risk for cessation of breastfeeding by 7 to 10 days of age. *Journal of Pediatrics, 141*, 659-664.

Hallowell, S.G., & Spatz, D.L. (2012). The relationship of brain development and breastfeeding in the late-preterm infant. *Journal of Pediatric Nursing, 27*, 154-162.

Hamilton, B.E., Martin, J.A., Osterman, M.J.K., & Rossen, L.M. (2019). *Births: Provisional data for 2018. Vital Statistics Rapid Release; no. 7.* Hyattsville, MD: National Center for Health Statistics.

Harris, D.L., Gamble, G.D., Weston, P.J., & Harding, J.E. (2017). What happens to blood glucose concentrations after oral treatment for neonatal hypoglycemia? *Journal of Pediatrics, 190*, 136-141.

Harris, D.L., Weston, P.J., Signal, M., Chase, J.G., & Harding, J.E. (2013). Dextrose gel for neonatal hypoglycemia (the Sugar Babies Study): A randomized, double-blind, placebo-controlled trial. *Lancet, 382*(9910), 2077-2083.

Hartmann, P.E., & Cregan, M. (2001). Lactogenesis and the effects of insulin-dependent diabetes mellitus and prematurity. *Journal of Nutrition, 131*, 3016S-3020S.

Hasegawa, J., Farina, A., Turchi, G., Zanello, M., & Baroncini, S. (2013). Effects of epidural analgesia on labor length, instrumental delivery, and neonatal short-term outcome. *Journal of Anesthesia, 27*, 43-47.

Hassan, B., & Zakerihamidi, M. (2018). The correlation between frequency and duration of breastfeeding and the severity of neonatal hyperbilirubinemia. *Journal of Maternal Fetal Neonatal Medicine, 31*, 457-463.

He, J.Q., Chen, B.Y., & Huang, T. (2008). Shanzhong acupoint treatment of postpartum hypogalactia: a multicenter randomized controlled study. *Chinese Acupuncture & Moxibustion, 28*, 317-320.

Hill, P.D., Aldag, J.C., & Chatterton, R.T. (1999). Effects of pumping style on milk production in mothers of non-nursing preterm infants. *Journal of Human Lactation, 15*, 209-216.

Hill P.D., Aldag J.C., Chatterton R.T., & Zinaman M. (2005). Comparison of milk output between mothers of preterm and term infants: the first 6 weeks after birth. *Journal of Human Lactation, 21*, 22–30.

Hobbs, A.J., Mannion, C.A., McDonald, S.W., Brockway, M., & Tough, S.C. (2016). The impact of caesarean section on breastfeeding initiation, duration and difficulties in the first four months postpartum. *BMC Pregnancy Childbirth, 16,* 90.

Hofer, M.A. (1994). Early relationships as regulators of infant physiology and behavior. *Acta Paediatrica, 397,* 9–18.

Hofer, M.A. (2005). The psychobiology of early attachment. *Clinical Neuroscience Research 4,* 291-300.

Hoover, K. (1998). Supplementation of newborn by spoon in the first 24 hours. *Journal of Human Lactation, 14,* 245.

Hubbard, E., Stellwagen, L., & Wolf, A. (2007). The late preterm infant: a little baby with big needs. *Contemporary Pediatrics,* November 1, 2007. Retrieved from https://health.ucsd.edu/specialties/obgyn/maternity/newborn/nicu/spin/staff/Documents/ContemporaryPediatricsThelatepreterminfant_AlittlebabywithbigneedsCME.pdf.

Huda, M.N., Lewis, Z.T., Kalanetra, K.M., Rashid, M., Ahmad, S.M., Raqib, R., Qadri, F., Underwood, M.A., Mills, D.A., & Stephensen, C.B. (2014). Stool microbiota and vaccine responses of infants. *Pediatrics, 134,* e362–e372.

Huff, K., Rose, R.S., & Engle, W.A. (2019). Late preterm infants: Morbidities, mortality, and management recommendations. *Pediatric Clinics of North America, 66,* 387-402.

Hurst, N., & Meier, P.P. (2005). Breastfeeding the preterm infant. In J. Riordan (Ed). *Breastfeeding and human lactation, 3rd Ed* (p. 376). Boston, MA: Jones and Bartlett Publishers.

## I

Inoue, N., Sakashita, R., & Kamegai, T. (1995). Reduction of masseter muscle activity in bottle-fed babies. *Early Human Development, 42,* 185-193.

Ize-Ilamu & Saheeb, 2011. Feeding intervention in cleft lip and palate babies: A practical approach to feeding efficiency and weight gain. *International Journal of Maxillofacial Surgery, 40,* 916-919.

## J

Jacobs, L.A., Dickinson, J.E., Hart, D.P., Doherty, D.A., & Faulkner, S.J. (2007). Normal nipple position in term infants measured on breastfeeding ultrasound. *Journal of Human Lactation, 23,* 52–59.

Jasani, B., Simmer, K., Patole, S.K., & Rao, S.C. (2017). Long chain polyunsaturated fatty acid supplementation in infants born at term. *Cochrane Database of Systematic Reviews 2017, Issue 3.* Art. No.: CD000376.

Jensen, D., Wallace, S., & Kelsay, P. (1994). LATCH: a breastfeeding charting system and documentation tool. *Journal of Obstetric, Gynecologic and Neonatal Nursing, 23,* 27-32.

Jiang, L.L. (2014). Observation on curative effect of 106 cases of postpartum hypogalactia treated by combination of TCM and Western Medicine. *Journal of Qilu Nursing, 20,* 124.

Jonsdottir, R.B., Jonsdottir, H., Skuladottir, A., Thorkelsson, T., & Flacking, R. (2020). Breastfeeding progression in late preterm infants from birth to one month. *Maternal Child Nutrition, 16,* e12893.

# K

Kair, L.R., Nidey, N.L., Marks, J.E., Hanrahan, K., Femino, L., Fernandez y Garcia, E., Ryckman, K., & Wood, K.E. (2020). Disparities in donor human milk supplementation among well newborns. *Journal of Human Lactation, 36,* 74-80.

Karl, D.J. (2004). Using principles of newborn behavioral state organization to facilitate breastfeeding. *American Journal of Maternal Child Nursing, 29,* 292-298.

Keith, D.R., Weaver, B.S., & Vogel, R.L. (2012). The effect of music-based listening interventions on the volume, fat content, and caloric content of breastmilk produced by mothers of premature and critically ill infants. *Advances in Neonatal Care, 12,* 112-119.

Kellams, A, Harrel, C., Omage, S., Gregory, C., Rosen-Carole, C., & the Academy of Breastfeeding Medicine. (2017). ABM clinical protocol #3: supplementary feedings in the healthy term breastfed neonate, revised 2017. *Breastfeeding Medicine, 12,* 188-198.

Kent, J.C., Gardner, H., & Geddes, D.T. (2016). Breastmilk production in the first 4 weeks after birth of term infants. *Nutrients, 8,* 756; doi:10.3390/nu8120756.

Kent, J.C., Geddes, D.T., Hepworth, A.R., & Hartmann, P.E. (2011). Effect of warm breastshields on breast milk pumping. *Journal of Human Lactation, 27,* 331-338.

Kent, J.C., Ramsay, D.T., Doherty, D., Larsson, M., & Hartmann, P.E. (2003). Response of breasts to different stimulation patterns of an electric breast pump. *Journal of Human Lactation, 19,* 179-187.

Kesaree, N., Banapurmath, C.R., Banapurmath, S., & Shamanur, K. (1993). Treatment of inverted nipples using a disposable syringe. *Journal of Human Lactation, 9,* 27-29.

Kuzniewicz, M.W., Parker, S-J., Schnake-Mahl, A., & Escobar, G.J. (2013). Hospital readmissions and emergency department visits in moderate preterm, late preterm, and early term infants. *Clinics in Perinatology, 40,* 753-775.

# L

Laptook, A., & Jackson, G. (2006). Cold stress and hypoglycemia in the late preterm ("near term") infant: Impact on nursery of admission. *Seminars in Perinatology, 30,* 24–27.

Law-Morstatt, L., Judd, D.M., Snyder, P., Baier, R.J., & Dhanireddy, R. (2003). Pacing as a treatment technique for transitional sucking patterns. *Journal of Perinatology, 23,* 483-488.

Lei, M., Liu, T., Li, Y., Liu, Y., Meng, L., & Jin, C. (2018). Effects of massage on newborn infants with jaundice: A meta-analysis. *International Journal of Nursing Science, 5,* 89-97.

Lober, A., Dodgson, J.E., & Kelly, L. (2020). Using the Preterm Infant Breastfeeding Behavior Scale (PIBBS) with late preterm infants. *Clinical Lactation, 11,* [ahead of print].

Loring, C., Gregory, K., Gargan, B., LeBlanc V., Lundgren, D., Reilly, J.....& Zaya, C. (2012). Tub bathing improves thermoregulation of the late preterm infant. *Journal of Obstetric, Gynecologic & Neonatal Nursing, 41,* 171-179.

Lu, P., Ye, ZQ, Qiu, J., Wang, XY, & Zheng, J.J. (2019). Acupoint-tuina therapy promotes lactation in postpartum women with insufficient milk production who underwent cesarean sections. *Medicine (Baltimore), 98,* e16456.

Ludington-Hoe, S.M., & Morgan, K. (2014). Infant assessment and reduction of sudden unexpected postnatal collapse risk during skin-to-skin contact. *Newborn and Infant Nursing Reviews, 14,* 28-33.

Ludwig, S.M., (2007). Oral feeding and the late preterm infant. *Newborn and Infant Nursing Reviews, 7,* 72-75.

# M

Makker, K., Alissa, R., Dudek, C., Travers, L., Smotherman, C., & Hudak, M.L. (2018). Glucose gel in infants at risk for transitional neonatal hypoglycemia. *American Journal of Perinatology, 35,* 1050-1056.

Mannel, R., & Peck, J.D. (2018). Outcomes associated with type of milk supplementation among late preterm infants. *Journal of Obstetric, Gynecologic, and Neonatal Nursing, 47,* 571-582.

Marasco, L., & West, D. (2020). *Making more milk, 2nd Ed.* New York: McGraw-Hill Education.

Marmet, C., & Shell, E. (1984). Training neonates to suck correctly. *MCN. The American Journal of Maternal Child Nursing, 9,* 401-407.

Martin, J.A., Hamilton, B.E., Osterman, M.J.K., & Driscoll, A.K. (2019). *Births: Final data for 2018. National Vital Statistics Reports; vol 68, no 13.* Hyattsville, MD: National Center for Health Statistics. Supplemental tables. Retrieved from: https://www.cdc.gov/nchs/data/nvsr/nvsr68/nvsr68_13_tables-508.pdf.

Matias, S.L., Dewey, K.G., Quesenberry, C.P., & Gunderson, E.P. (2014). Maternal prepregnancy obesity and insulin treatment during pregnancy are independently associated with delayed lactogenesis in women with recent gestational diabetes mellitus. *American Journal of Clinical Nutrition, 99,* 115-121.

Mazurek, T., Mikiel-Kostyra, K., Mazur, J., Wieczorek, P., Radwanska, B., & Pachuta-Wegier, L. (1999). Influence of immediate newborn care on infant adaptation to the environment. *Medycyna Wieku Rozwojowego, 3,* 215-224.

McDowell, K.M., Jobe, A.H., Fenchel, M., Hardie, W.D., Gisslen, T., Young, L.R., Chougnet, C.A., Davis, S.D., & Kallapur, S.G. (2016). Pulmonary morbidity in infancy after exposure to chorioamnionitis in late preterm infants. *Annals of the American Thoracic Society, 13,* 867-876.

McEwen, B.S., & Seeman, T. (1999). Protective and damaging effects of mediators of stress. Elaborating and testing the concepts of allostasis and allostatic load. *Annals of the New York Academy of Sciences, 896,* 30–47.

McLaurin, K.K., Hall, C.B., Jackson E.A., Owens, O.V., & Mahadevia, P.J. (2009). Persistence of morbidity and cost differences between late-preterm and term infants during the first year of life. *Pediatrics, 123,* 653-659.

Medoff-Cooper, B., Holditch-Davis, D., Verklan, M.T., Fraser-Askin, D., Lamp, J., Santa-Donato, A., Onokpise, B., Soeken, K.L., & Bingham, D. (2012). Newborn clinical outcomes of the AWHONN late preterm infant research-based practice project. *Journal of Obstetric, Gynecologic and Neonatal Nursing, 41,* 774-785.

Meier, P. (1988). Bottle- and breastfeeding: Effects on transcutaneous oxygen pressure and temperature in preterm infants. *Nursing Research, 37,* 36-41.

Meier, P.P., Furman, L.M., & Degenhardt, M. (2007). Increased lactation risk for late preterm infants and mothers: Evidence and management strategies to protect breastfeeding. *Journal of Midwifery and Women's Health, 52,* 579-587.

Miller, V., & Riordan, J. (2004). Treating postpartum breast edema with areolar compression. *Journal of Human Lactation, 20,* 223-226.

Mirzaie, P., Mohammad-Alizadeh-Charandabi, S., Goljarian, S., Mirghafourvand, M., & Hoseinie, M.B. (2018). The effect of foot reflexology massage on breast milk volume of mothers with premature infants: A randomized controlled trial. *European Journal of Integrative Medicine, 17*(suppl C), 72-78.

Mizuno, K., Nishida, Y., Mizuno, N., Taki, M., Murase, M., & Itabashi, K. (2008). The important role of deep attachment in the uniform drainage of breastmilk from mammary lobe. *Acta Paediatrica, 97,* 1200-1204.

Mobbs, E.J., Mobbs, G.A., & Mobbs, A.E. (2016). Imprinting, latchment and displacement: A mini review of early instinctual behavior in newborn infants influencing breastfeeding success. *Acta Paediatrica, 105,* 24-30.

Mohammadpour, A., Valiani, M., Sadeghnia, A., & Talakoub, S. (2018). Investigating the effect of reflexology on the breast milk volume of preterm infants' mothers. *Iranian Journal of Nurse Midwifery Research, 23,* 371-375.

Moore, E.R., Bergman, N., Anderson G.C., & Medley, N. (2016). Early skin-to-skin contact for mothers and their healthy newborn infants. *Cochrane Database Systematic Reviews, 11*:CD003519.

Moral, A., Bolibar, I., Seguranyes, G., Ustrell, J., Sebastia, G., Martinez-Barba, C., & Rios, J. (2010). Mechanics of sucking: comparison between bottle feeding and breastfeeding. *BMC Pediatrics, 10*(6). doi: 10.1186/1471-2431-10-6.

Moreira, C.M.D., Cavalcante-Silva, R.P.G.V., Jujinaga, C.I., & Marson, F. (2017). Comparison of the finger-feeding versus cup feeding methods in the transition from gastric to oral feeding in preterm infants. *Journal de Pediatria (Rio J), 93,* 585-591.

Morgan, B.E., Horn, A.R., & Bergman, N.J. (2011). Should neonates sleep alone? *Biological Psychiatry, 70,* 817–825.

Morrison, B., Ludington-Hoe, S., & Anderson, G.C. (2006). Interruptions to breastfeeding dyads on postpartum day 1 in a university hospital. *Journal of Obstetric, Gynecologic, and Neonatal Nursing, 35,* 709-716.

Morton, J., Hall, J.Y., Wong, L., Thairu, L., Benitz, W.E., & Rhine, W.D. (2009). Combining hand techniques with electric pumping increases milk production in mothers of preterm infants. *Journal of Perinatology, 29,* 757-764.

# N

Natarajan, G., & Shankaran, S. (2016). Short- and long-term outcomes of moderate and late preterm infants. *American Journal of Perinatology, 33,* 305-317.

Neubauer, S.H., Ferris, A.M., Chase, C.G., Fanelli, J., Thompson, C.A., Lammi-Keefe, C.J.,...& Green, K.W. (1993). Delayed lactogenesis in women with insulin-dependent diabetes mellitus. *American Journal of Clinical Nutrition, 58,* 54-60.

Newton, M., & Newton, N.R. (1948). The let-down reflex in human lactation. *Pediatrics, 33,* 698-704.

Nicholson, W.L. (1993). The use of nipple shields by breastfeeding women. *Australian College of Midwives Incorporated Journal, 6,* 18-24.

Nilsson, U. (2009). Soothing music can increase oxytocin levels during bed rest after open-heart surgery: a randomized control trial. Journal of Clinical Nursing, 18, 2153-2161.

Nommsen-Rivers, L.A. (2016). Does insulin explain the relationship between maternal obesity and poor lactation outcomes? An overview of the literature. *Advances in Nutrition, 7,* 407-414.

Nyqvist, K.H. (2008). Early attainment of breastfeeding competence in very preterm infants. *Acta Paediatrica, 97,* 776-781.

Nyqvist, K.H., Farnstrand, C., Eeg-Olofsson, K.E., & Ewald, U. (2001). Early oral behaviour in preterm infants during breastfeeding: An electro-myographic study. *Acta Paediatrica, 90,* 658-663.

Nyqvist, K.H., Rubertsson, C., Ewald, U., & Sjoden, P.O. (1996). Development of the preterm infant breastfeeding behavior scale (PIBBS): A study of nurse-mother agreement. *Journal of Human Lactation, 12,* 207-219.

# O

Ostfeld, B.M., Schwartz-Soicher, O., Reichman, N.E., Teitler, J.O., & Hegyi, T. (2017). Prematurity and sudden unexpected infant deaths in the United States. *Pediatrics, 140,* e20163334.

Ottolini, K.M., Andescavage, N., Kapse, K, Basu, S., & Limperopoulos, C. (2019). Breastfeeding boosts metabolites important for brain growth. Science-Daily. *ScienceDaily, 27* April 2019. Retrieved from: www.sciencedaily.com/releases/2019/04/190427104808.htm.

# P

Pados, B.F., Park, J., Thoyre, S.M., Estrem, H., & Nix, W.B. (2016). Milk flow rates from bottle nipples used after hospital discharge. *MCN American Journal of Maternal Child Nursing, 41,* 237-243.

Palmer, M.M. (1993). Identification and management of the transitional suck pattern in premature infants. *Journal of Perinatal and Neonatal Nursing, 7,* 66-75.

Parker, L.A., Sullivan, S., Krueger, C., & Mueller, M. (2015). Association of timing of initiation of breastmilk expression on milk volume and timing of lactogenesis stage II among mothers of very low-birth-weight infants. *Breastfeeding Medicine, 10,* 84-91.

Penny, F., Judge, M., Brownell, E., & McGrath, J.M. (2018a). What is the evidence for use of a supplemental feeding tube device as an alternative supplemental feeding method for breastfed infants? *Advances in Neonatal Care, 18,* 31-37.

Penny, F., Judge, M., Brownell, E., & McGrath, J.M. (2018b). Cup feeding as a supplemental, alternative feeding method for preterm breastfed infants: An integrative review. *Maternal Child Health Journal, 22,* 1568-1579.

Perrine, C.G., Scanlon, K.S., Li, R., Odom, E., & Grummer-Strawn, L.M. (2012). Baby-Friendly hospital practices and meeting exclusive breastfeeding intention. *Pediatrics, 130,* 54-60.

Phillips, R.M., Goldstein, M., Hougland, K., Nandyal, R., Pizzica, A., Santa-Donato, A., Staebler, S., Stark, A.R., Treiger, T.M., & Yost, E., on behalf of The National Perinatal Association. (2013). Multidisciplinary guidelines for the care of late preterm infants. *Journal of Perinatology, 33(Suppl 2), S5–S22.*

Pike, M., Kritzinger, A., & Kruger, E. (2017). *Breastfeeding characteristics of late-preterm infants in a kangaroo mother care unit. Journal of Human Lactation, 12,* 637-644.

Premji, S.S., Currie, G., Reilly, S., Dosani, A., Oliver, L.M., Lodha, A.K., & Young, M. (2017). A qualitative study: Mothers of late preterm infants relate their experiences of community-based care. *PLoS One, 12*(3), e0174419.

Preusting, I., Brumley, J., Odibo, L., Spatz, D.L., & Louis, J.M. (2017). Obesity as a predictor of delayed lactogenesis II. *Journal of Human Lactation, 33,* 684-691.

# R

Radtke, J.V. (2011). The paradox of breastfeeding-associated morbidity among late preterm infants. *Journal of Obstetric, Gynecologic, and Neonatal Nursing, 40,* 9-24.

Raju, T.N., Higgins, R.D., Stark, A.R., & Leveno, K.J. (2006). Optimizing care and outcome for late-preterm (near-term) infants: A summary of the workshop sponsored by the National Institute of Child Health and Human Development. *Pediatrics, 118,* 1207-1214.

Rampono, J., Simmer, K., Ilett, K.F., Hackett, L.P., Doherty, D.A., Elliot, R., Kok, C.H., Coenen, A., & Forman, T. (2009). Placental transfer of SSRI and SNRI antidepressants and effects on the neonate. *Pharmacopsychiatry, 42,* 95–100.

Ramsay, D.T., Kent, J.C., Owens, R.A., & Hartmann, P.E. (2004). Ultrasound imaging of milk ejection in the breast of lactating women. *Pediatrics, 113,* 361-367.

Ramsay, D.T., Mitoulas, L.R., Kent, J.C., Cregan, M.D., Doherty, D.A., Larsson, M., & Hartmann, P.E. (2006). Milk flow rates can be used to identify and investigate milk ejection in women expressing breast milk using an electric breast pump. *Breastfeeding Medicine, 1,* 13-23.

Rasmussen, K.M., & Kjolhede, C.L. (2004). Prepregnant overweight and obesity diminish the prolactin response to suckling in the first week postpartum. *Pediatrics, 113,* e465-e471.

Rautava, S., Luoto, R., Salminen, S., & Isolauri, E. (2012). Microbial contact during pregnancy, intestinal colonization and human disease. *Nature Reviews Gastroenterology and Hepatology, 9,* 565-576.

Riddle, S.W., & Nommsen-Rivers, L.A. (2016). A case-control study of diabetes during pregnancy and low milk supply. *Breastfeeding Medicine, 11,* 80-85.

Rocha, N.M., Martinez, F.E., & Jorge, S.M. (2002). Cup or bottle for preterm infants: Effects on oxygen saturation, weight gain, and breastfeeding. *Journal of Human Lactation, 18,* 132-138.

Rommel, N., Van Wijk, M., Boets, B., Hebbard, G., Haslam, R., Davidson, G., & Omari, T. (2011). Development of pharyngo-esophageal physiology during swallowing in the preterm infant. *Neurogastroenterology & Motility, 23,* e401-e408.

Romond, M-B., Colavizza, M., Mullié, C., Kalach, N., Kremp, O., Mielcarek, C., Izard, D. (2008). Does the intestinal bifidobacterial colonisation affect bacterial translocation? *Anaerobe, 14,* 43–48.

Rose, R., & Engle, W.A. (2017). Optimizing care and outcomes for late preterm neonates. *Current Treatment Options in Pediatrics, 3,* 32-43.

## S

Salisbury, A.L., O'Grady, K.E., Battle, C.L., Wisner, K.L., Anderson, G.M., Stroud, L.R., Miller-Loncar, C.L., Young, M.E., & Lester, B.M. (2016). The roles of maternal depression, serotonin reuptake inhibitor treatment, and concomitant benzodiazepine use on infant neurobehavioral functioning over the first postnatal month. *American Journal of Psychiatry, 173,* 147-157.

Santoro Jr, W., Martinez, F.E., Ricco, R. G., & Jorge, S.M. (2010). Colostrum ingested during the first day of life by exclusively breastfed healthy newborn infants. *Journal of Pediatrics, 156,* 29-32.

Schneider, L.W., Crenshaw, J. T., & Gilder, R.E. (2017). Influence of immediate skin-to-skin contact during cesarean surgery on rate of transfer of newborns to NICU for observation. *Nursing for Women's Health, 21,* 28-33.

Schytt, E., Lindmark, G., & Waldenstrom, U. (2005). Physical symptoms after childbirth: prevalence and associations with self-rated health. *BJOG: An International Journal of Obstetrics and Gynecology, 112,* 210-217.

Sengupta, S., Carrion V., Shelton, J., Wynn, R.J., Ryan, R.M., Singhal, K., & Lakshminrusimha, S. (2013). Adverse neonatal outcomes associated with early-term birth. *JAMA Pediatrics, 167,* 1053-1059.

Simonson, C., Barlow, P., Dehennin, N., Sphel, M., Toppet, V., Murillo, D., & Rozenberg, S. (2007). Neonatal complications of vacuum-assisted delivery. *Obstetrics and Gynecology, 109,* 626-633.

Slattery, J., Morgan, A., & Douglas, J. (2012). Early sucking and swallowing problems as predictors of neurodevelopmental outcome in children with neonatal brain injury: A systematic review. *Developmental Medicine and Child Neurology, 54,* 796-806.

Stephenson, T., Budge, H., Mostyn, A., Pearce, S., Webb, R., & Symonds, M.E. (2001). Fetal and neonatal adipose tissue maturation: A primary site of cytokine and cytokine-receptor action. *Biochemical Society Transactions, 29,* 80-85.

Stellwagen, L.M., Hubbard, E., & Wolf, A. (2007). The late preterm infant: a little baby with big needs. *Contemporary Pediatrics,* November 1, 2007.

Stewart, D.L., Barfield, W.D., & Committee on Fetus and Newborn. (2019). Updates on an at-risk population: Late-preterm and early-term infants. *Pediatrics, 144*, e20192760.

Symonds, M.E. (2013). Brown adipose tissue growth and development. *Scientifica, 2013*, Article ID 305763. http://dx.doi.org/10.1155/2013/305763

Symonds, M.E., Mostyn, A., Pearce, S., Budge, H., & Stephenson, T. (2003). Endocrine and nutritional regulation of fetal adipose tissue development. The Journal of Endocrinology, 179, 293-299.

## T

Thorley, V. (1997). Cup feeding: Problems created by incorrect use. *Journal of Human Lactation, 13*, 54-55.

Thoyre, S.M., & Carlson, J. (2003a). Occurrence of oxygen desaturation events during preterm infant bottle-feeding near discharge. *Early Human Development, 72*, 25-36.

Thoyre, S.M., & Carlson, J.R. (2003b). Preterm infants' behavioural indicators of oxygen decline during bottle-feeding. *Journal of Advanced Nursing, 43*, 631-641.

Tilstra, A.M. & Masters, R.K. (2020). *Worth the weight? Recent trends in obstetric practices, gestational age, and birth weight in the United States.* Demography, [ahead of print] https://doi.org/10.1007/s13524-019-00843-w

Tozier, P.K. (2013). Colostrum versus formula supplementation for glucose stabilization in newborns of diabetic mothers. *Journal of Obstetric, Gynecologic, and Neonatal Nursing, 42*, 619-628.

Turcksin, R., Bel, S., Galjaard, S., & Devlieger, R. (2014). Maternal obesity and breastfeeding intention, initiation, intensity and duration: A systematic review. *Maternal Child Nutrition, 10*, 166–183.

## V

Valdez, J., Lujan, C., & Valdez, M. (2018). Effects of kinesio tape application on breastmilk production [poster]. *Breastfeeding Medicine, 13*(S2), S36.

## W

Walker, M. (2008). Breastfeeding the late preterm infant. *Journal of Obstetric, Gynecologic & Neonatal Nursing, 37*, 692–701.

Walker, M. (2016). Nipple shields: What we know, what we wish we knew, and how best to use them. *Clinical Lactation, 7*, 100-107.

Walsh, J.M., Doyle, L.W., Anderson, P.J., Lee, K.J., & Cheong, J.L. (2014). Moderate and late preterm birth: Effect on brain size and maturation at term-equivalent age. *Radiology, 273*, 232-240.

Wang, B. (2009). Sialic acid is an essential nutrient for brain development and cognition. *Annual Review of Nutrition, 29*, 177-222.

Wang, H.C., An, J.M., & Han, Y. (2007). Acupuncture for the treatment of postpartum hypogalactia: A multicenter randomized controlled study. *Chinese Acupuncture & Moxibustion, 27*, 85-88.

Whyte, R.K., & Canadian Paediatric Society, Fetus and Newborn Committee. (2010). Safe discharge of the late preterm infant. *Paediatric Child Health, 15*, 655-660.

Wiberg-Itzel, E., Pembe, A.B., Wray, S., Wihlback, A-C., Darj, E,. Hoesli, I., & Akerud, H. (2014). Level of lactate in amniotic fluid and its relation to the use of oxytocin and adverse neonatal outcome. *Acta Obstetricia et Gynecologica Scandinavica, 93*, 80–85.

Widstrom, A-M., Brimdyr, K., Svensson, K., Cadwell, K., & Nissen, E. (2019). Skin-to-skin contact the first hour after birth, underlying implications and clinical practice. *Acta Paediatrica, 108*, 1192-1204.

Widstrom, A-M., Brimdyr, K., Svensson, K., Cadwell, K., & Nissen, E. (2020). A plausible pathway of imprinted behaviors: Skin-to-skin actions of the newborn immediately after birth follow the order of fetal development and intrauterine training of movements. Medical Hypotheses, 134, 109432.

Widstrom, A-M., Lilja, G., Aaltomaa-Michalias, P., Dahllof, A., Lintula M., & Nissen, E. (2011). Newborn behavior to locate the breast when skin-to-skin: A possible method for enabling early self-regulation. *Acta Paediatrica, 100*, 79-85.

Wight, N., Marinelli, K.A., & The Academy of Breastfeeding Medicine. (2014). ABM protocol #1: guidelines for blood glucose monitoring and treatment for hypoglycemia in term and late-preterm neonates, revised 2014. *Breastfeeding Medicine, 9*, 173-179.

Wilson-Clay, B., & Hoover, K. (2002). *The breastfeeding atlas.* Austin, TX: LactNews Press.

Wolf, L.S., & Glass, R.P. (1992). *Feeding and swallowing disorders in infancy: assessment and management.* Austin, TX: ProEd.

Wolf, L.S., & Glass, R.P. (2013). The Goldilocks problem: milk flow that is not too fast, not too slow, but just right or, why milk flow matters and what to do about it. In C.W. Genna (Ed.). *Supporting sucking skills in breastfeeding infants, 2nd Ed.* (pp. 149-170). Burlington, MA: Jones and Bartlett Learning.

Woythaler, M. (2019). Neurodevelopmental outcomes of the late preterm infant. *Seminars in Fetal and Neonatal Medicine, 24*, 54-59.

# X

Xian, D. (2017). Application of acupuncture therapy in nursing care of maternal lack of breast milk. *Nursing Research of China, 31*, 2301-2303.

# Y

Yigit, F., Cigdem, Z., Temizsoy, E., Cingi, M.E., Korel, O., Yildirim, E., & Ovali, F. (2012). Does warming the breasts affect the amount of breastmilk production? *Breastfeeding Medicine, 7,* 487-488.

Yilmaz, G., Caylan, N., Karacan, C.D., Bodur, I., & Gokcay, G. (2014). Effect of cup feeding and bottle-feeding on breastfeeding in late preterm infants: A randomized controlled study. *Journal of Human Lactation, 30,* 174-179.

Yu, X., Li, J., Lin, X., & Luan, D. (2019). Association between delayed lactogenesis II and early milk volume among mothers of preterm infants. *Asian Nursing Research (Korean Society of Nursing Science), 13,* 93-98.

# Z

Zangen, S., Di Lorenzo, C., Zangen, T., Mertz, H., Schwankovsky, L., & Hyman, P.E. (2001). Rapid maturation of gastric relaxation in newborn infants. *Pediatric Research, 50,* 629-632.

Zhao, J., Gonzalez, F., & Mu, D. (2011). Apnea of prematurity: From cause to treatment. *European Journal of Pediatrics, 170,* 1097-105.

Zhou, H-y, Li, L., Li, D., Li, X., Meng, H-j, Gao, X-m, Jiang, H-j, Cao, L-r, & Zhu, Y-l. (2009). Clinical observation on the treatment of post-cesarean hypogalactia by auricular points, sticking-pressure. *Chinese Journal of Integrative Medicine, 15,* 117-120.

# About the Author

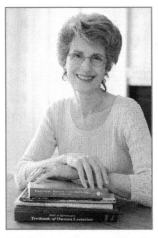

**Marsha Walker, RN, IBCLC** is a registered nurse and international board certified lactation consultant (IBCLC). She has been assisting breastfeeding families in hospital, clinic, and home settings since 1976. Marsha is the executive director of the National Alliance for Breastfeeding Advocacy (NABA). NABA is the US IBFAN organization that monitors the International Code of Marketing of Breastmilk Substitutes in the United States. As such, she advocates for breastfeeding at the state and federal levels. She served as a vice president of the International Lactation Consultant Association (ILCA) from 1990-1994 and in 1999 as president of ILCA. She is a previous board member of the US Lactation Consultant Association, Baby Friendly USA, and the Massachusetts Breastfeeding Coalition. She serves as USLCA's representative to the USDA's Breastfeeding Promotion Consortium, NABA REAL's representative to the US Breastfeeding Committee, Associate Editor of Clinical Lactation, and a board member of the Massachusetts Lactation Consultant Association. Marsha is an international speaker, and an author of numerous publications including ones on the hazards of infant formula use, Code issues in the US, and *Breastfeeding Management for the Clinician: Using the Evidence, 5th edition.*

Made in the USA
Columbia, SC
03 August 2020